Gemmotherapy For Our Animal Friends

Stephen R. Blake, DVM, CVA, CVH

"The Pet Whisperer"

in collaboration with Pam Fettu, CCH, RSHom (NA)

First Edition January 2011.

ISBN: 978-0-615-43847-4

Contents

Contents 3

Disclaimer 7

Forward.. 8

Dedication.. 10

Preface 12

Introduction 19

Acute and Chronic Conditions 23

Method of Dosing...................................... 25

Physical Exam Checklist for Pets 27

Common Ailments 40

    ACNE.. 40

    AGGRESSION & RABIES MIASM 44

    ARTHRITIS... 46

    AURAL HEMATOMAS.............................. 51

    BITES & STINGS 54

    BLOAT.. 57

    BURNS & SCALDS 59

    CONJUNCTIVITIS................................... 60

CONVULSIONS (SEIZURES) 63

COUGHING 65

CYSTITIS 69

DECAYING OR ABSESSED TEETH 73

DEGENERATIVE MYELOPATHY....................74

DIABETES MELLITUS..................................76

DIARRHEA...78

DISCHARGE FROM THE VULVA 80

DOG & CAT BITES......................................82

EAR INFECTIONS 85

EAR MITES..88

FEAR OF NOISES 90

FOOD & GARBAGE POISONING 92

FLY STRIKE...95

FOXTAILS & FOREIGN BODIES...................97

GINGIVITIS & MOUTH INFLAMMATION.......99

HEART DISEASE 101

HIP DYSPLASIA 103

HOTSPOTS 105

HYPOPYON (EYE PROBLEMS) 108

INFECTIONS 110

INTERVERTEBRAL DISC DISEASE (SLIPPED DISC)112

ITCHING 114

KIDNEY FAILURE 118

LIVER DISORDER 120

MANGE 122

NOSEBLEED.. 124

OVERHEATING 125

POSTPARTUM CONDITIONS 127

PROSTATE AFFECTIONS......................... 129

RANULA 131

RETAINED TESTICLE (CRYPTORCHIDISM) 133

RINGWORM... 134

SKIN INFECTIONS & ERUPTIONS 136

SNAKE BITES 140

SNEEZING AND NASAL CONGESTION ... 142

SPONDYLITIS.. 144

SPRAINS & STRAINS 146

THYROID DISEASE (Hyperthyroidism) 148

THYROID DISEASE (Hypothyroidism) 150

URINARY INCONTINENCE 152

VOMITING 154

Draining and Detoxification.....................................156

Gemmotherapy Remedies - Common Name 159

Gemmotherapy Remedies - Botanical Name 182

Gemmotherapy Materia Medica 205

Common Conditions and the Gemmotherapy Remedies
Used to Treat Them 218

Most Frequently Used Gemmotherapy Remedies in the
Care of Animals..236

Resources 238

Suggested Reading...254

Disclaimer

These statements have not been evaluated by the FDA and are not intended to be a substitute for professional medical advice. Nor is this information meant to diagnose, treat, cure, or prevent any disease. It is meant for educational purposes.

Stephen R. Blake, DVM, CVH, CVA
San Diego, California, USA

Forward

Dr. Steve Blake has been a good friend and a mentor since I first met him almost two decades ago. As one of the pioneers in veterinary holistic health, he has incessantly sought new ways to help the four-footed ones, and probably even the crawlers, fliers, and swimmers, to whom we dedicate our lives and practices.

I have been hearing Dr. Steve talk about gemmotherapies for a few years now. Like many, at first I wondered if these were remedies made from rubies and emeralds and such, but no, they are homeopathically prepared herbal tinctures, most commonly from plant buds. The root "gemmo" is from the Latin for bud. I finally began using Gemmotherapy remedies, using some of the information on Dr. Steve's web site, and finally studying more on my own. I have seen some very nice results in my patients, and I am grateful that I finally paid attention to my good friend.

Now, you too can incorporate these remedies into your "toolkit" for helping animal companions, whether for those who live with you or for your patients. *Gemmotherapy for Our Animal Friends* provides a solid information base to start you on a path to success. The book is succinct, yet it covers many conditions that affect animals, and Dr. Steve's instructions will get you going in a flash.

May your animals and you benefit from the love and wisdom you will find within these pages.

Don Hamilton, DVM
Author of *Homeopathic Care for Cats and Dogs: Small Doses for Small Animals*

Dedication

I want to thank all of my many teachers, both human and animal, for hanging in there with me through thick and thin. If it were not for my best friend, my lovely wife Charene, my life as I know it today would never have come to pass. Her belief in me and my work has made it possible for me to get to this point in my life where I can share my journey with all who wish to listen. I want to thank my sons Sean and Scott, for being a wonderful part of my life and for being kind to humans and animals alike. My five grandchildren, Tanner, Nicholas, Madison, Skylar and Dr. Christian make my heart smile with the loving footprints they leave on my heart each and every day. In memory of my Father, Stephen, my Mother, Marie and my Spiritual Mother, Helen, I want them to know how much they continue to help me on my journey for inner consciousness and happiness for myself and all I am fortunate to be with. Thank you all for caring.

Thank you, Pam Fettu, my friend and fellow Homeopath (of the human kind) for being the motivation for completing this work. She is a wonderful collaborator and caring person for animals and people alike. Thank you Pam for all you did to make this project a success.

I also want to thank Dr. Bera Dordoni, my friend and editor of my newsletter *The Pet Whisperer* for editing my book. She is a great friend to me and our animal friends.

Preface

How it Began

This is my journey through life, which would never have happened if I had not become a veterinarian. As a child, I wanted to be a doctor and help "fix" people. I was fascinated by science, biology, mathematics, physics and fixing things. When I got into my second year of premed, I realized it wasn't for me. After telling a classmate that I was going to drop out, he said, "Why don't you become a veterinarian?" The rest is history.

That change in my life made it possible for me to witness unconditional love for the past 30 years. The animals saved my life and are my reason for writing this book. To them I owe more than I can ever repay.

In the beginning of my veterinary career, I practiced medicine as best I could with the tools I learned at Colorado State University School of Veterinary Medicine. As the years rolled by, I began to question if what I had been taught was all there was to help animals.

In the early 1980s I got ill, and I was lucky to find a homeopathic physician, Dr. Dorin Gutu, who diagnosed pesticide toxicity. His advice was to stop being a veterinarian, wear rubber gloves or die. The gloves lasted about one patient and I knew that wasn't going to work. I asked (actually demanded) that all my clients not use pesticides on their pets, or I couldn't treat them.

To my amazement I got busier than ever! I realized I had to learn new methods for caring for animals if chemicals were out. Where was I going to find this training? The answer came quickly. I met a fellow veterinarian, Dr. Carvel Tiegert, at a conference where he asked me a simple question: "Do you think vitamins are important in treating animals?" I answered "yes" and he put me on a quest to learn as much as I could about alternative medicine.

I have been certified by the Homeopathic Veterinary Academy as a Homeopathic Veterinarian and as a Veterinary Acupuncturist by the International Veterinary Acupuncture Society. I mainly use Aromatherapy, Classical Homeopathy, Bach Flowers, Gemmotherapy, Massage, Acupuncture and Nutrition to care for my patients. I have found that ninety-five percent of time I am able to help animals with their medical needs without using drugs or surgery. The use of drugs and surgery has a place in veterinary medicine but their need is much less than we are led to believe.

The Greek definition of physician is teacher and that is what I do my very best to do when caring for my animal friends. I have been practicing integrative veterinary medicine for over 27 years and found it to be the most satisfying time of my career as a veterinarian. Any time someone tells me that that these alternatives will not work on animals, I respond with one of my favorite quotes that I found in a box of ginger snaps long ago.

The person who says it cannot be done should not interrupt the person doing it!

Chinese Proverb

This quote and others throughout the book have helped guide my approach to living my life and caring for my friends, the animals. What I would like to leave with all of you is this —the animal kingdom knows all of this and far more. WE are the students in the classroom of nature and our teachers are the animals. Respect your teachers and apply what they teach you. To do any less is to show disrespect for the only teachers I know that have as their sole purpose unconditional love for all life, no matter what it looks like. If the world would come together in this collective consciousness, there would be world peace. To this theme I dedicate this book.

My Dream

I have had a dream, a vision and desire to see mankind reach the spiritual level of a dog. I know you are asking yourselves, why a dog? First of all DOG is GOD spelled backward, which should give you a little hint as to where I am going with this stream of consciousness. I have known in my heart that my animal friends are here as teachers for all humans to learn about living in the *now, consciousness* and *being present.*

I have spent thousands of hours teaching pet owners how to be more proactive in the health care of their pets. That has been my goal with each ear that will lean in my direction and will listen to me and my friends, the animals, to make us all aware of our roles as teacher and steward of the animals and the planet. Taking on these roles is a blessing for each of us.

I have often said to my caregivers, friends, readers, family, etc. "The only blight on the planet is man." History proves we have done more harm to the planet than any other species in the history of the world. Our collective unconsciousness has devastated plants and animals alike at an alarming exponential rate.

However, my dear friends the animals, have unending patience. They show me with their unconditional love, which is their only response toward this blight, that there is hope and all we have to do is get out of the way and

15

follow the teachings of the plants and animals. Stop. Look. Listen. Not to your latest technological wonder, but to the nature of life in the plant or animal closest to you. Simply put, be *happy,* and to accomplish this collective *happiness,* all we have to do is be *compassionate* for all that is.

As I always say to my caregivers and readers, when you are faced with a challenge: "Be a dog, be a cat, be a horse." By following this simple statement, mankind will truly be *in the moment, collectively conscious and present, in the collective conscious of now.* Be a dog today and show unconditional love for all that is.

My Gratitude to My Friends the Animals

It has been an honor to serve all the animals and their caregivers that have come into my life. I have been truly blessed with the kindest clients a veterinarian could ever ask for. As I always say, "I love treating all animals; it's the caregivers who can be a challenge."

The *smile* the animals put on my heart is a gift that can never be fully repaid. All I can do is to continue to pay forward what they have taught and continue to teach me, with the passing of each day, to all who will listen. All I ask of anyone who hears my words is to please share them with all you know and ask them to do the same. I call this paying it forward and if we all do this; the world will be a *heaven* on *earth*.

Albert, Elmo and Dr. Louie

Albert and Elmo, two of my best friends—two wonderful Basset hounds, who were my best teachers and assistants for 14½ and 13 years respectively. I know we will meet again when it is my time to cross the Rainbow Bridge and join them once again on our eternal journey serving others. These two great spirits taught me the meaning of being "The Pet Whisperer" and inspired this book. They taught me patience and how to listen to their friends, the animals. They are with me now in spirit as they were in body before they crossed the Rainbow Bridge. My Watsons, as I was their Sherlock Holmes.

Dr. Louie, the only Canine Veterinarian in the world, is my new best friend and assistant. He came into my life as did Albert and Elmo, just when I needed help on my journey through the laboratory of life.

Dr. Louie is truly a gift that keeps giving. He reminds me, with the passing of each day, how important it is to be in the moment and enjoy *living*. Life is living and all the animals live life. Their wish for us is to do the same. Let us lend them our ear.

Our ability to reach unity in diversity will be the beauty and test of our children.

Gandhi

Introduction

My first introduction to Gemmotherapy was back in the early 1980's when I was blessed with hearing Dr. Max Tetau speak on the subject in United States at an Orthomolecular meeting. He spoke in French and had a translator who made it possible for me to get the basics about this amazing healing modality. I had never heard of Gemmotherapy and was unable to get it in the United States at that time. I was very impressed with his knowledge and made a promise to myself when the time was right, I would study more about this amazing drainage system and incorporate it into my practice. Years went by and in the 1990's I was reintroduced to Gemmotherapy and the rest is history. I use it in all my patients and have found it to be an integral part in helping the animals heal themselves optimally.

Gemmotherapy is a drainage system developed in Europe over 40 years ago. Preliminary research on using plant buds therapeutically was started by Dr. Pol Henry of Belgium in the 1950s. After extensive clinical research on immature plant materials, Max Tetau, M.D., introduced the therapeutic technique known as Gemmotherapy some twenty years later.

The process begins when the buds and young shoots of the immature plants are macerated and extracted with glycerin for twenty-one days then made into a 1X potency (1 part extract in 9 parts water). These extracts are high in growth factors, which contain the phyto-hormones, auxins and gibberellins. These active ingredients are present in the buds, but begin to disappear as the plant matures. Auxins have a fetal hormonal action, which is found only in the buds of plants. Gibberellins stimulate RNA and protein synthesis. Gibberellins are also only present in the buds and not in the whole plant. Researchers have found, by utilizing this process releases, the greatest amount of healing potential from the plants.

There are presently over sixty commercially available Gemmotherapy remedies. Each of these plant extracts has very specific actions on every living organism.

The main principle behind Gemmotherapy is drainage and detoxification of the organism at the cellular level.

By completing this process, only then can the body truly heal itself. Drainage works by increasing the ability of the organs of elimination, known as the emunctories, to remove toxic wastes from the body. When toxins build up, the body will do its best to release them from the cells and tissues, through pathways called emunctories. These emunctories include the kidney and bladder (through urine), intestines (through stool), uterus (through menstruation), skin (through perspiration, lungs (through deep breathing), and the liver. Although the liver does not lead to the outside of the body, it is the main detoxifying organ in the body. Nearly everything in the body filters through the liver at least once. Many of the environmental toxins to which your animals are exposed, such as flea and tick repellents, household insecticides, drugs, antibiotics, vaccines, heavy metals and other carcinogenic chemicals, are converted in the liver. Here, the liver does its best to remove these toxins through the cellular processes, excreting them through the emunctories.

I have utilized classical homeopathy, acupuncture, glandular therapy, nutrition, aromatherapy and Bach flowers for nearly 20 years. Many times the animals were not progressing to a healthy state no matter what I tried; there was a factor none of my treatments could remedy. It wasn't until I discovered Gemmotherapy that I was able to help these otherwise 'incurables.'

By no means am I suggesting this system is a cure-all because there is no such animal that I have discovered in 30 years of searching for one. I am sharing with you another tool that can complement any treatments you are presently utilizing, including conventional systems of surgery and pharmaceuticals.

Acute and Chronic Conditions

If your pet has an "acute" condition, meaning a condition which has just 'happened,' it usually comes on suddenly and it doesn't repeat itself, (unless the animal exposes itself to the same allergen again and again). There's a cause and effect reaction. Examples of acute conditions are . . . your pet gets sprayed with pepper spray, eats a poisonous substance, or suffers a trauma.

However, when the symptom is seen repeatedly, such as a chronic eye, ear, or nasal discharge; chronic itching, continually licking the feet, scooting, eating dirt, sticks, or foreign materials (known as pica), then the condition is not acute, it is chronic. In other words, a "chronic" condition is a symptom that continually repeats itself.

In a chronic condition, the animal may be predisposed to this condition and it comes on and repeats itself again and again,. This is a sign of chronic disease. You treat the condition and it comes back, you treat it again, and once more it comes back. Hairballs in cats are a sign of chronic gastrointestinal problems. Other "chronic" conditions include: crusty dryness on the bridge of the nose, thickening of the pads, or repeated diarrhea or vomiting (more than once or twice a year).

Most conditions I deal with in pets are of a chronic nature. So, remember, when you are treating your pet, determine first if the symptom is acute or chronic.

Method of Dosing

Using Gemmotherapy remedies for your animals can be started along with your other programs with a complementary effect. It's important to note, the dosage you give is individualized according to the animal's individual energy level and how sensitive the animal is to the environment.

Chronic, debilitated cases should be started out very slowly with between 1 to 5 drops once a day. If you have an ultra-sensitive animal, mix **one** drop of the Gemmotherapy remedy in a half cup spring water and give **just one drop of this mixture once until you are comfortable with the reaction**.

Reduce the amount of water and gradually increase the dose of the remedy until you've reached 5 drops per day with no adverse reaction. At this point if there are no more symptoms of the original disease state, stop and go to a maintenance dose of 5 drops once per week as a preventive aspect of the program.

The best way I've found to administer the drops of remedy are:

1. Place the drops right on the animal's food.

2. Onto the animal's nose; or massage into the hairless part of the ear.

3. In a separate bowl of clean, filtered water specifically for the remedy.

Sensitivity Levels:

Level 1- Very Sensitive: The animal is easily affected by change in diet, weather, environmental changes, traveling, changing of routine. Give 1 drop of remedy, or dilute as described above.

Level 2- Average: This animal has more chronic problems, with occasional flare-ups, like itching and scratching, small hot spots, nothing of a severe origin. Give 3 drops of remedy.

Level 3- Bullet Proof: This animal has a strong constitution; itches a lot, scoots often, some discharge from the eyes and ears, but has no chronic problems. Give 5 drops of remedy.

Physical Exam Checklist for Pets

Authored by: The VIN Emergency Medicine Staff

www.veterinarypartner.com

To identify an illness or abnormal situation, you must first be able to recognize what is normal for your pet. Below you will find a quick checklist to determine what is normal. The primary suggestion is to give your pet a "mini" physical exam occasionally when there is nothing wrong so you get used to what is normal for your pet. A hands-on physical exam in the comfort of your pet's home is the best way to learn what is normal for your pet. Record the normal values at the back of this chapter.

APPEARANCE:

Before starting the hands-on exam, stand back and look at your pet for a few minutes. Their posture, breathing, activity level, and general appearance can tell you a lot.

Now start the physical exam, making sure to look at the following areas. Consult a veterinarian if an abnormal condition exists or you are concerned about any exam findings.

NOSE

❏ Normal

- Moist and clean

- Smooth surface

- Uniformed pigmentation

❏ Abnormal

- Crusts on bridge of nose and on wings of nostrils

- Dry or cracked nose

- Nasal discharge (such as thick greenish mucus)

- Bleeding

- Depigmentation

SKIN- Feel your pet's skin and hair/coat, noting any masses or sores.

❏ Normal

- Shiny and smooth hair/coat

- Soft and unbroken skin

- Minimal odor

☐ Abnormal

- Sparse or patchy hair/coat

- Open sores or scabs

- Oily or dirty feeling to coat

- Foul or rancid odor

- Dander

EYES

☐ Normal

- Bright, moist, and clear; centered between the eyelids; pupils equal in size

- Whites of the eye should not appear colored (such as red or yellow) and should have only a few visible blood vessels

- Pupils shrink equally when bright light is shined into either eye; pupils enlarge equally when the eyes are held closed or the room darkened.

☐ Abnormal

- Dull, sunken eyes; eyes that appear dry; thick discharge from eyes; one or both eyes not centered

- Pupils unequal in size

- Pay close attention to the color of the whites of your pet's eyes. Abnormal colors that indicate problems are yellow (jaundice), or red (bloodshot)

- Pupils fail to respond or respond differently when bright light is shined into either eye; pupils fail to respond or respond differently to the dark

EARS

Chronic ear problems are common in pets, and are often a result of allergies to inhaled pollen (like hay fever in people) that are then complicated by secondary infections with bacteria or fungus. Ear infections can be painful and head shaking can lead to an accumulation of blood (or hematoma) in the floppy part of the ear called the pinna.

☐ Normal

- Your pet's ears should be clean and odor-free

- Skin smooth and without wounds

- Clean and dry

- Almost odor-free

- Typical carriage for breed; pain-free

☐ Abnormal:

- Wounds or scabs on skin

- Lumps or bumps on skin

- Any sign of rash

- Crust, moisture, or other discharge in ear canal

- Any strong odor from the ear

- Atypical carriage for breed; for example, a droopy ear in a breed with normally erect ears

- Painful or swollen ears.

MOUTH

Press on the gum tissue with your finger or thumb and release quickly. Watch the color return to the gums. This checks the capillary refill time (CRT) and is a crude assessment of how well the heart and circulatory system are working. A normal CRT is 1 to 2 seconds for color to return. This can be a difficult test to interpret sometimes (for example, if your pet has dark or pigmented gums), and should not be relied upon as definitive evidence that your pet is sick or healthy.

❏ Normal

- Teeth are clean and white; gums are uniformly pink.

❏ Abnormal

- Tartar accumulation around the base of the teeth

- The gums are red, pale, inflamed, or sore in appearance

- Offensive odor

NECK/CHEST/BREATHING

It is difficult to hear a pet breathe at all except when they are panting.

❏ Normal

- The chest wall moves easily to and fro during respiration; most of the act of breathing is performed by the chest wall

❏ Abnormal

- Any unusual noise heard while the pet is breathing could indicate a problem, especially if the noise is new for the pet.

- There is noticeable effort by the pet to move the chest wall.

- The abdomen is actively involved in the act of inhaling and exhaling.

ABDOMEN (Stomach)

Touch and feel (palpate) the stomach. Start just behind the ribs and gently press your hands into the abdomen, feeling for abnormalities. If your pet has just eaten, you may be able to feel an enlargement in the left part of the abdomen just under the ribs. Proceed toward the rear of the body, passing your hands gently over the abdomen.

☐ Normal:

- No lumps, bumps, or masses

- No discomfort on palpation

- No distension of the abdominal wall

☐ Abnormal:

- Any lump, bump, or mass may be abnormal.

- Palpation causes groaning or difficulty breathing. Any evidence or indication of pain is a serious finding. Use caution to avoid being bitten

- The abdomen feels hard or tense and it appears distended

- Any pain felt during an abdominal palpation could be a problem. Consult your veterinarian

- Excessive sounds from abdomen and/or flatulence

SKIN TURGOR

The skin turgor test may be the most helpful one to determine whether an animal is well hydrated. This test can be affected by several factors other than hydration status, such as weight loss, age and general skin condition, but it can help you make a rough determination of your pet's hydration status. To perform this test, pull the skin over the chest or back into a tent and release it quickly; avoid the skin of the neck as it's often too thick for this test. Observe the skin as it returns to its resting position.

☐ Normal:

- The skin snaps back into position quickly.

❏ Abnormal

- The skin returns slowly or remains slightly tented. This is a sign of possible dehydration.

PULSE & HEART RATE

Learn to locate the pulse on your pet before a crisis. The best place on a cat or dog is the femoral artery in the groin area. Place your fingers around the front of the hind leg and move upward until the back of your hand meets the abdominal wall. Move your fingertips back and forth on the inside of the thigh until you feel the pulsing sensation as the blood rushes through the artery. Count the number of pulses in 15 seconds and multiply by 4. This will give you the pulse rate in beats per minute (BPM). Pulse rate is a highly variable finding and can be affected by recent exercise, excitement or stress. Do not use the heart rate at the sole evidence that your pet is sick or healthy.

❏ Normal: Pulse is easily palpated, strong, and regular

- Cats: 100 to 160 beats per minute (bpm). A relaxed cat may have a slower pulse.
- Small dogs: 90 to 130 bpm

- Medium dogs: 70 to 110 bpm
- Large/giant dogs: 60 to 100 bpm. A relaxed dog may have a slower pulse.

❏ Abnormal

- Too rapid or too slow
- Pulse is weak, irregular, or hard to locate.

TEMPERATURE

Taking your pet's temperature is an easy and important procedure and can be done with a digital thermometer. Digital thermometers are easier to read and can be inexpensively purchased at a pharmacy.

Rectal temperatures are more accurate than axillary (between the front leg and the body) temperatures. Lubricate the thermometer with petroleum jelly. Gently and slowly insert the thermometer into the rectum about 1 or 2 inches. If it does not slide in easily, do not force it. Leave it in for 2 minutes, then read and record the temperature.

❏ Normal

- Temperature is between 101°F and 102.5°F

- The thermometer is almost clean when removed.

☐ Abnormal

- Temperature is below 100°F or above 103°F

- There is evidence of blood, diarrhea, or black, tarry stool on the thermometer

It may be easier to take your cat's temperature if you have someone to help you. Do not risk taking your pet's temperature if you feel there is a risk of being bitten.

A Final Note

Know the "normal values" for your pet. Record the results of your pet's home examination using the outline below. Watch your pet closely so you know when something is wrong. Become familiar with these normal values before a crisis so you can recognize an abnormal finding.

Normal Values for my Pet

My pet _____

has the following normal values:

Normal Weight: _____pounds

Resting Heart Rate (Pulse): _____
beats per minute

Resting Respiratory Rate: _____
breaths per minute

Rectal Temperature: _____
degrees Fahrenheit

Normal Gum Color: _____

Normal Whites of the Eyes: _____

"Knowledge is acquired through study,

wisdom through observation"

Unknown

Common Ailments

ACNE

Acne in dogs and cats is a sign of chronic disease and should be treated as such. By that, I mean it is a symptom of a deeper issue in the body manifesting itself on the surface of the body in the region of the chin area. You want to avoid using any cortisone, antifungal or antibiotics on these areas or giving any of these drugs orally. Although this will temporarily palliate or make the symptoms disappear, and you might find this seems to bring relief to the animal, in reality these drugs drive the issue at hand deeper and suppress the healing of the animal.

SIGNS & SYMPTOMS

- Black Discharge from Skin on Chin
- Eruption on Chin
- Itching
- Swelling

TREATMENT

I recommend keeping the area clean if necessary to help the animal be comfortable. If the patient is uncomfortable you use the following:

- Calendula Tincture: Mix 1 drop of Calendula tincture, per ounce of spring water. Rinse the area after cleaning with this tincture.

and/or

- Rescue Remedy Tincture: Mix 1 drop Rescue Remedy per ounce of water. Massage into the area as needed for discomfort.

Both of these products **will not** suppress the healing process and allow the healing to progress with the least amount of discomfort.

I recommend that the dog or cat be put on **Common Juniper** (to detoxify and strengthen the liver and kidneys).

- **Common Juniper**

  Cats: 3 to 5 drops of **Common Juniper** once per day for a total of 6 weeks

Dogs: 3 to 5 drops of **Common Juniper** once per day
          for a total of 6 weeks

After the six weeks is completed, take this same above
dosage, 3 to 5 drops, once per week thereafter to
detoxify and strengthen the liver and kidneys. Beginning
each spring, repeat the six-week spring-cleaning
protocol once again.

If the symptoms gets worse or the skin is itchy, **STOP**
the **Common** Juniper and do not repeat until the
cleansing effect subsides and then resume. You may
have to stop and start many times until the animal has
sufficiently removed the toxins which are being released
by the **Common Juniper**. Keep track of the days on
and off the **Common Juniper.** Your goal is six weeks in
total for the cleanse to be effective.

- **European Walnut and Rye Grain**

   Cats: 1 to 3 drops of **European Walnut** and **Rye Grain** per day

   Dogs: 5 to 10 drops of **European Walnut** and **Rye Grain** per day

I recommend using **European Walnut** and **Rye Grain** as the two main remedies for helping the animals heal from within.

If the condition gets worse, stop all three and wait for the area to clear. Once the detoxifying healing clears, repeat the sequence again. Stop and start as the animal indicates until they are completely healed.

AGGRESSION & RABIES MIASM

I recommend that you never vaccinate, use flea or tick chemicals, or heartworm medication on cats and dogs who have aggression issues or on any animals that have any aggressive tendencies.

SIGNS & SYMPTOMS

- Impulsive Attack Behavior
- Sudden Behavior Changes
- Sudden Desire To Bite
- Usually Worse After Vaccination With Rabies
- Worse with Noise or Movement People or Dog Aggression Unprovoked

TREATMENT

I recommend **Black Currant, Common Birch and Lime Tree** at the below dosage twice per day or as needed for seizures. Once there are no further symptoms, I dose weekly thereafter to help detoxify.

- **Black Currant, Common Birch,** and **Lime Tree**

    Cats: 3 to 5 drops of each, twice per day or as needed for seizures

Dogs: 3 to 5 drops of each, twice per day or as needed for seizures

I recommend putting all animals on **Common Juniper** at the below dosage for a total of six weeks.

- **Common Juniper**

    Cats: 3 to 5 drops of **Common Juniper** once per day for a total of 6 weeks

    Dogs: 3 to 5 drops of **Common Juniper** once per day for a total of 6 weeks

After the six weeks is completed, take this same above dosage, 3 to 5 drops, once per week thereafter to detoxify and strengthen the liver and kidneys.

Beginning each spring, repeat the six week spring-cleaning protocol once again.

ARTHRITIS

Sadly, in this day and age, this is a very common issue in all ages of dogs, cats and horses. The main cause is chronic inflammation of the joints. Living beings need to dig their toes or heels or foot pads into the earth for at least a few hours a day. If you are an animal caregiver, then both you and your animal(s) need to find some dirt, grass, ocean, beaches, rocks, stone tile on concrete, or concrete and get your bare feet (or paws) directly onto one or more of them daily. All of these are conductors and will insure they are keeping the electrical balance of you and your animal's bodies in check. The grounding effect helps to remove the positive charge that builds up in our bodies due to free radical formation secondary to metabolism, cell repair and replacement, EMF, alternating current in the walls of homes, repeater towers and transmitters, high voltage electrical power lines, Wi-Fi and cell phone transmissions. If it is affecting you, it is surely affecting your animal. You can read about this on my web site
www.thepetwhisperer.com.

Vaccines, chemicals, herbicides, pesticides, drugs, water, stress and, poor diet can be etiologies. Avoid all of these extrinsic factors as much as you can!

SIGNS & SYMPTOMS

- Pain In Joints
- Sensitive to Touch
- Swelling

TREATMENT

I recommend that you give all animals with arthritis **Common Birch.** This is the universal drainer for the body, good for the liver, the joints, and great for helping reduce inflammation anywhere in the body.

- **Common Birch**

  Cats: 1 to 3 drops, twice per day
  Dogs: 5 to 10 drops, twice per day
  Horses: 5 to 10 drops, twice per day

For knees, elbows and shoulder joints I recommend **Wild Woodvine.**

- **Wild Woodvine**

  Cats: 1 to 3 drops, twice per day
  Dogs: 5 to 10 drops, twice per day
  Horses: 5 to 10 drops, twice per day

If you have a giant breed puppy, start them all off at 8 weeks of age with this remedy to help them develop the healthiest joints possible during their early development.

For hip joints I recommend *both* **Common Birch** and **Wild Woodvine**.

Common Birch is especially good for hip dysplasia in that it helps the circulation and regeneration of the entire hip complex.

- **Common Birch and Wild Woodvine**

  Cats: 1 to 3 drops of each, twice per day
  Dogs: 5 to 10 drops of each, twice per day
  Horses: 5 to 10 drops of each, twice per day

If small joints are involved (toes, wrists and ankles), I recommend **Common Birch, Wild Woodvine** and **European Grape Vine (**this remedy is excellent for arthritis of small joints).

- **Common Birch, Wild Woodvine and European Grape Vine**

  Cats: 1 to 3 drops of each, twice per day
  Dogs: 5 to 10 drops of each, twice per day
  Horses: 5 to 10 drops of each, twice per day

For issues of the spine, (Spondylosis, Disc Disease, wobblers, and back pain), I recommend using **Common Birch, Wild Woodvine** and **Mountain Pine.** The jingle to remember is: "Mountain Pine straightens your spine."

- **Common Birch, Wild Woodvine and Mountain Pine**

  Cats: 1 to 3 drops of each, twice per day
  Dogs: 5 to 10 drops of each, twice per day
  Horses: 5 to 10 drops of each, twice per day

I recommend putting all animals on **Common Juniper** at the below dosage for a total of six weeks.

- **Common Juniper**

  Cats: 3 to 5 drops of **Common Juniper** once per day for a total of 6 weeks
  Dogs: 3 to 5 drops of **Common Juniper** once per day for a total of 6 weeks

After the six weeks is completed, take this same above dosage, 3 to 5 drops, once per week thereafter to detoxify and strengthen the liver and kidneys. Beginning each spring, repeat the six-week spring-cleaning protocol once again.

If the symptoms gets worse or the skin is itchy, **STOP** the **Common** Juniper and do not repeat until the cleansing effect subsides and then resume. You may have to stop and start many times until the animal has sufficiently removed the toxins which are being released by the **Common Juniper**. Keep track of the days on and off the **Common Juniper.** Your goal is six weeks in total for the cleanse to be effective.

AURAL HEMATOMAS

This is a common condition found mainly in dogs but I have seen a few cats with this condition. This is NOT a trauma issue. This is an immune issue. It is a sign of chronic disease and needs to be managed as such. I would recommend getting an integrative veterinarian who understands chronic-disease-management protocols. Through the years I have avoided having to perform surgery ninety-five percent of the time in both cats and dogs using homeopathy and gemmotherapy treatment. Work with a homeopathic veterinarian along with what I have written below to avoid unnecessary drugs and surgery. .

Many decades ago I learned that, if you do nothing, the ear will completely heal in about four weeks. I know this sounds hard to believe, but that is what I have observed. The end result is a scar-crinkled ear flap which you'll get, even with surgery.

SIGNS & SYMPTOMS

- Drooping of Ear with Swelling
- Shaking of Head
- Sudden Onset
- Swelling of Ear Flap

The main remedies for this condition are **Rowan Tree** and **Black Currant.**

- **Black Currant and Rowan Tree**

  Cats: 1 to 3 drops of each, twice per day
  Dogs: 5 to 10 drops of each, twice per day
  Horses: 5 to 10 drops of each, twice per day

I recommend that the dog, horse or cat be put on **Common Juniper** (to detoxify and strengthen the liver and kidneys).

- **Common Juniper**

  Cats: 3 to 5 drops of **Common Juniper** once per day for a total of 6 weeks

  Dogs: 3 to 5 drops of **Common Juniper** once per day for a total of 6 weeks

  Horses: 3 to 5 drops of **Common Juniper** once per day for a total of 6 weeks

After the six weeks is completed, take this same above dosage, 3 to 5 drops, once per week thereafter to detoxify and strengthen the liver and kidneys. Beginning each spring, repeat the six-week spring-cleaning protocol once again.

If the symptoms gets worse or the skin is itchy, **STOP** the **Common Juniper** and do not repeat until the cleansing effect subsides and then resume. You may have to stop and start many times until the animal has sufficiently removed the toxins which are being released by the **Common Juniper**. Keep track of the days on and off the **Common Juniper**. Your goal is six weeks in total for the cleanse to be effective.

BITES & STINGS

Insect bites, such as fleas, spiders, flies and ticks are the most common insects our pets encounter in their daily lives. Prevention is the best medicine. You can read about natural ways to prevent fleas and ticks on my web site www.thepetwhisperer.com .

Clean water, natural foods and fresh air are the basics for staying healthy and naturally repelling fleas, ticks and other parasites. Stay away from excessive vaccinations and chemicals of any kind.

SIGNS & SYMPTOMS

- Itching
- Painful To Touch
- Redness
- Swelling

TREATMENT

If your dog is bitten by a flea, spider, fly or tick, I recommend the following course of action:

1. Clean the bite with a mild soap and water. (Lavender shampoo from Young Living Essential Oils is recommended http://thepetwhisperer.com/essential_oil.html)

2. Make a solution of:

   1 drop of **Black Currant** and **1** drop of **Rye Grain** per ounce of water.

   Put this solution directly on the bite. Repeat this every 15 minutes until the animal is no longer bothered by the wound.

3. At the same time, give the following Gemmotherapy remedies orally every 15 minutes until the animal is no longer bothered by the wound.

- **Black Currant**

  Cats: 1 to 3 drops every 15 minutes
  Dogs: 5 to 10 drops every 15 minutes
  Horses: 5 to 10 drops every 15 minutes

BLOAT

This is a condition mainly found in dogs. There are many theories on what causes it, but the main thing to remember is this symptom signifies that there is a good chance you're looking at a chronic disease. You should have an integrative veterinarian help you with the management of this condition. If you suspect bloat is the issue, seek emergency veterinary assistance due to the threat of death secondary to this condition. **Vaccines are one of the main triggers of this condition** and for this reason, never vaccinate an animal once they have had an episode of bloat.

SIGNS & SYMPTOMS

- Abdominal Distention
- Abnormal Salivating
- Dry Heaving
- Restlessness
- Lethargy
- Rapid Heart Rate
- Signs of Discomfort

TREATMENT

Give **Fig Tree, Black Currant** and **Wine Berry** acutely, every 15 minutes until the dog is not showing any symptoms of bloat. Once there are no more symptoms, fast the dog for 24 hours, except for liquids, and gradually add solid food when the animal is stable.

- **Fig Tree, Black Currant** and **Wine Berry**

  Dogs: 5 drops of each, every 15 minutes

BURNS & SCALDS

This is a rare issue in animals but when it happens it can be very painful. I have found the best topical agent is the **essential oil lavender.** I recommend putting one drop of essential oil to one ounce of water and mist the area as often as needed for comfort and healing. You can find lavender under Essential Oils, on my web site: http://thepetwhisperer.com/essential_oil.html

SIGNS & SYMPTOMS

- Erosion of Skin
- Painful Blistering
- Sloughing of Skin

TREATMENT

- **European Alder and Black Currant**

  Cats: 1 to 3 drops of each, twice per day
  Dogs: 5 to 10 drops of each, twice per day
  Horses: 5 to 10 drops of each, twice per day

Give these two Gemmotherapy remedies daily until the area is healed.

CONJUNCTIVITIS

This is a very common symptom of dogs, cats and horses. This is an inflammatory condition of the tissues around the globe of the eye. The main causes are topical irritants, allergic reactions to substances (pollen, chemicals, herbicides, pesticides, vaccines and drugs topically applied or orally). How best to treat this condition? Avoid exposing your pet to any of the above substances when possible.

SIGNS & SYMPTOMS

- Discharge
- Itching
- Redness
- Swelling

TREATMENT

The eyes are the windows to the liver in Traditional Chinese Medicine (TCM) and for that reason I recommend always treating the liver when there are problems with the eyes.

I recommend putting all animals on **Common Juniper** at the above dosage for a total of six weeks.

- **Common Juniper**

  Cats: 3 to 5 drops of **Common Juniper** once per day for a total of 6 weeks

  Dogs: 3 to 5 drops of **Common Juniper** once per day for a total of 6 weeks

  Horses: 3 to 5 drops of **Common Juniper** once per day for a total of 6 weeks

After the six weeks is completed, take this same above dosage, 3 to 5 drops, once per week thereafter to detoxify and strengthen the liver and kidneys.

Beginning each spring, repeat the six-week spring-cleaning protocol once again.

I also recommend **Black Currant** as needed for inflammation of the conjunctiva.

- **Black Currant**

    Cats: 1 to 3 drops four times per day, orally, as need for inflammation

    Dogs: 5 to 10 drops four times per day, orally, as need for inflammation

    Horses: 5 to 10 drops four times per day, orally, as need for inflammation

CONVULSIONS (SEIZURES)

This is a condition seen mainly in dogs and rarely in cats. I recommend that you never vaccinate, use flea or tick chemicals or heartworm medication on animals who have ever had a seizure of any magnitude.

SIGNS & SYMPTOMS

- Collapse with Spasm of Limbs
- Head Tremors
- Involuntary Spasms of The Nervous System
- Involuntary Thrashing of Legs
- Staring

TREATMENT

- **Black Currant, Common Birch and Lime Tree**

  Dogs: 3 to 5 drops of each, twice a day or as
          needed for seizures

I recommend **Black Currant, Common Birch** and **Lime Tree** dosed twice per day or as needed for seizures. Once there are no further symptoms, I dose once a week thereafter to (3-5 drops) to help detoxify and strengthen the animal's resistance to further seizures.

I also recommend **Common Juniper**

- **Common Juniper**

  Cats: 3 to 5 drops of **Common Juniper** once
  per day for a total of 6 weeks

  Dogs: 3 to 5 drops of **Common Juniper** once
  per day for a total of 6 weeks

  Horses: 3 to 5 drops of **Common Juniper** once per
  day for a total of 6 weeks

After the six weeks is completed, take this same above dosage, 3 to 5 drops, once per week thereafter to detoxify and strengthen the liver and kidneys.

Beginning each spring, repeat the six-week spring-cleaning protocol once again.

COUGHING

If the cough is an acute issue (meaning it hasn't occurred repeatedly prior to using the Gemmotherapy remedies), you would first use **Lithy Tree.** If you do not see any improvement in the cough after an hour, add **Fig Tree.** If after another hour there still is no change, add **European Walnut.** If you are still not seeing any change in the cough after a few hours, seek veterinary care. As long as the Gemmotherapy remedies are helping the animal improve, continue with treatment. If this is not the case, time to see the veterinarian.

If the cough is a chronic cough, I recommend using **Lithy Tree** and **European Walnut**

SIGNS & SYMPTOMS

- Episodes Breathing with Difficulty
- Hard Breathing
- Hard Expectoration

- **Lithy Tree**

    Cats: 1 to 3 drops every 15 minutes until you see a change in the frequency and intensity and then repeat only as needed.

    Dogs: 5 to 10 drops every 15 minutes until you see a change in the frequency and intensity and then repeat only as needed.

    Horses: 5 to 10 drops every 15 minutes until you see a change in the frequency and intensity and then repeat only as needed.

- **Fig Tree**

    Cats: 1 to 3 drops every 15 minutes until you see a change in the frequency and intensity and then repeat only as needed.

    Dogs: 5 to 10 drops every 15 minutes until you see a change in the frequency and intensity and then repeat only as needed.

Horses: 5 to 10 drops every 15 minutes until you
see a change in the frequency and
intensity and then repeat only as needed.

- **European Walnut**

  Cats: 1 to 3 drops every 15 minutes until you
  see a change in the frequency and
  intensity and then repeat only as needed.

  Dogs: 5 to 10 drops every 15 minutes until you
  see a change in the frequency and
  intensity and then repeat only as needed.

  Horses: 5 to 10 drops every 15 minutes until you
  see a change in the frequency and
  intensity and then repeat only as needed.

If the cough is a **chronic cough**, I recommend the
following:

- **Lithy Tree and European Walnut**

  Cats: 1 to 3 drops of each every 15 minutes until
  you see a change in the frequency and

intensity. Repeat only as needed, for a maximum of three days.

Dogs: 5 to 10 drops of each every 15 minutes until you see a change in the frequency and intensity. Repeat only as needed, for a maximum of three days.

Horses: 5 to 10 drops of each every 15 minutes until you see a change in the frequency and intensity. Repeat only as needed, for a maximum of three days.

Remember, once you see improvement only repeat the remedies if the dog or cat coughs. If you do not see any improvement in the cough within three days, seek veterinary care.

CYSTITIS

This is more of a problem in cats, especially male cats, but it does occur in dogs and horses. In my opinion one of the main triggers of inflammation of the bladder is vaccines. If your pet has a history of bladder or kidney issues, NEVER vaccinate due to the risk secondary to repeated vaccinations in these patients. You can read about vaccination protocols and dangers of vaccination on my web site **www.thepetwhisperer.com**

SIGNS & SYMPTOMS

- Frequent Urination
- Incomplete Efforts to Urinate
- Pain with Urination
- Urgency to Urinate

TREATMENT

Male Cats

In male cats you have to be extremely careful that he is not obstructed. If you are not sure, seek veterinary assistance right away. Usually an obstructed male cat is very ill and lethargic. I would recommend all male cat owners have their veterinarians or veterinary technician show them how to palpate a normal bladder and what to feel for if they are obstructed.

Once you are confident he is not obstructed, you can start the male cat on the following Gemmotherapy treatment.

Male Cats: 3 drops of **Common Juniper** every time he tries to urinate.

If you do not see improvement in six repeated treatments add in 3 drops of **Black Currant.**

If you do not see improvement in six repeated treatments of 3 drops **Common Juniper** and 3 drops **Black Currant** to help reduce the swelling in the urethra and or bladder, seek veterinary care.

However, if he begins to urinate normally, continue treating with 3 drops of **Common Juniper** every time he urinates

If you notice he's having some difficulty, repeat again (3 drops of **Common Juniper**) as needed.

I have found that by doing the above treatment in male cats, I have not had to recommend or catheterize a male cat or perform a perineal urethrostomy.

Female Cats

In female cats, treat the same way but you do not need to worry about obstruction issues due to the difference in their anatomies. Ninety-five percent of urinary tract infections are sterile, so antibiotics are not needed in the vast majority of these cases.

Dogs and Horses

In dogs and horses, I recommend **Common Juniper and Silver Birch**.

> Dogs: 5 to 10 drops of **Common Juniper** each time the dog attempts to urinate.

> Horses: 5 to 10 drops of **Common Juniper** each time the horse attempts to urinate.

Abnormal urination includes frequent attempts to urinate small amounts of urine, straining to urinate, or blood in the urine. As long as you see the animal improving with each dose of the remedy, you are safe to continue.

If you do not see any improvement with 5 or 6 doses of the **Common Juniper**, add in **Silver Birch**.

Dogs: 5 to 10 drops of **Common Juniper** and **Silver Birch** each time the dog attempts to urinate.

Horses: 5 to 10 drops of **Common Juniper** and **Silver Birch** each time the horse attempts to urinate..

As long as you see your dog or horse improving (needing less of the remedies, less often, you are doing fine). If this is not the case, off to the veterinarian for further help.

DECAYING OR ABSESSED TEETH

This is mainly an issue in dogs and cats. You should seek the care of a veterinarian for determining which teeth need extraction and the need for antibiotics in treating the infection.

SIGNS & SYMPTOMS

- Odor
- Painful When Eating
- Redness of Gums
- Swelling

TREATMENT

- **Common Birch**

    Cats: 1 to 3 drops every day until veterinarian care is received

    Dogs: 4 to 10 drops every day until veterinarian care is received

DEGENERATIVE MYELOPATHY

This is most often seen in dogs but does occur in cats as well. The forming of bone spurs along the ventral aspect of the spinal column is a result of chronic inflammation and instability of the spine.

SIGNS & SYMPTOMS

- Gradual Paralysis of Hind Limbs
- Painless Dragging of Back Feet
- Progressive Weakness in Rear Legs
- Wobbly Rear Legs When Standing or Walking

TREATMENT

- **Mountain Pine, Black Currant, Giant Redwood and Common Birch.**

    Cats: 3 to 5 drops of each, twice per day
    Dogs: 3 to 5 drops of each, twice per day

Once there are no further symptoms, I dose weekly thereafter to help detoxify and strengthen the spine.

I recommend putting all animals on **Common Juniper** at the below dosage for a total of six weeks.

- **Common Juniper**

    Cats: 3 to 5 drops of **Common Juniper** once
             per day for a total of 6 weeks

    Dogs: 3 to 5 drops of **Common Juniper** once
             per day for a total of 6 weeks

After the six weeks is completed, take this same above dosage, 3 to 5 drops, once per week thereafter to detoxify and strengthen the liver and kidneys.

Beginning each spring, repeat the six-week spring-cleaning protocol once again.

DIABETES MELLITUS

This is more common in dogs and cats than horses. I have never treated a horse with diabetes, but if I had one as a patient, I would treat it just like a cat. I always have said a horse is a cat in a horse suit because they are so sensitive to chemicals and vaccines just like cats.

I put all my diabetics on a grain-free diet, no vaccines or chemicals of any kind and suggest they try massaging the pads of the animal's feet with an organic essential oil, **Ginger**. This is an excellent essential oil for diabetics and helps to regulate blood sugars.

SIGNS & SYMPTOMS

- Excessive Appetite with Weight Loss
- Excessive Thirst
- Excessive Urination
- Sugar in Urine

TREATMENT

I recommend you put them on **European Walnut** and **Hedge Maple.**

- **European Walnut and Hedge Maple**

  Cats: 1 to 3 drops of each, twice per day
  Dogs: 5 to 10 drops of each, twice per day
  Horses: 5 to 10 drops of each, twice per day

I recommend putting all animals on **Common Juniper** at the below dosage for a total of six weeks.

- **Common Juniper**

  Cats: 3 to 5 drops of **Common Juniper** once per day for a total of 6 weeks

  Dogs: 3 to 5 drops of **Common Juniper** once per day for a total of 6 weeks

  Horses: 3 to 5 drops of **Common Juniper** once per day for a total of 6 weeks

After the six weeks is completed, take this same above dosage, 3 to 5 drops, once per week thereafter to detoxify and strengthen the liver and kidneys. Beginning each spring, repeat the six-week spring-cleaning protocol once again.

DIARRHEA

This is a very common issue in animals and can often be chronic in nature. If you do not see any improvement in three days or less with the following treatment, seek veterinary help.

Fasting is the first step, with the exception of water. Start the dog or cat on **Fig Tree.** Repeat this each time the animal has diarrhea. If you do not see this helping within three treatments, add **Wine Berry** at the same dose regiment. If after three treatments you still do not see any improvement, add **European Walnut.** As long as you see improvement and resolution of the diarrhea within 72 hours, your friend will do just fine. If this is not the case, off to the local veterinarian for further assessment.

SIGNS & SYMPTOMS

- Increased Frequency of Loose-to-Watery Stools
- Unable to Control Release of Stools

TREATMENT

- **Fig Tree**

  Cats: 1 to 3 drops of **Fig Tree**
  Dogs: 5 to 10 drops of **Fig Tree**
  Horses: 5 to 10 drops of **Fig Tree**

If you do not see this helping within three treatments, add **Wine Berry** at the same dose regiment.

  Cats: 1 to 3 drops of **Fig Tree** and **Wine Berry**
  Dogs: 5 to 10 drops of **Fig Tree** and **Wine Berry**
  Horses: 5 to 10 drops of **Fig Tree** and **Wine Berry**

If after three treatments, you still do not see any improvement, add **European Walnut.**

  Cats: 1 to 3 drops of **Fig Tree** and **Wine Berry** and **European Walnut**
  Dogs: 5 to 10 drops of **Fig Tree** and **Wine Berry** and **European Walnut**
  Horses: 5 to 10 drops of **Fig Tree** and **Wine Berry** and **European Walnut**

If the diarrhea is **not** resolved within 72 hours, seek veterinary care for your pet.

DISCHARGE FROM THE VULVA

Discharge from the vulva is usually caused by infection of vaginal area or of the uterus. Vaccines can trigger this condition and for that reason I recommend not vaccinating dogs with any discharge from the vaginal area. I recommend **Raspberry, Common Birch** and **Giant Redwood** to treat this ailment.

SIGNS & SYMPTOMS

- Green, yellow or clear or creamy discharge from vulva
- Odor
- Redness, and or itching
- Sticky hair around vulva
- Swelling of vulva

TREATMENT

- **Common Birch, Giant Redwood** and **Raspberry**

    Cats: 1 to 3 drops of each, twice per day until there is no longer any discharge present. Dose once weekly at the same dose for prevention.

Dogs: 5 to 10 drops of each, twice per day until there is no longer any discharge present. Dose once weekly at the same dose for prevention.

Horses: 5 to 10 drops of each, twice per day until there is no longer any discharge present. Dose once weekly at the same dose for prevention.

I recommend putting all animals on **Common Juniper** at the below dosage for a total of six weeks.

- **Common Juniper**

    Cats: 3 to 5 drops of **Common Juniper** once per day for a total of 6 weeks

    Dogs: 3 to 5 drops of **Common Juniper** once per day for a total of 6 weeks

    Horses: 3 to 5 drops of **Common Juniper** once per day for a total of 6 weeks

After the six weeks is completed, take this same above dosage, 3 to 5 drops, once per week thereafter, to detoxify and strengthen the liver and kidneys.

DOG & CAT BITES

Dog or cat bites are very painful for the animals and should be seen by a veterinarian to assess the need for surgery or conventional medical care. You must always be very careful with animals that have been bitten. They generally are in pain and may bite you if you unintentionally hurt them in your attempt to help them.

To be safe, you should use a muzzle or wrap them in a towel to help prevent being bitten by the injured animal. If you are not confident in a situation like this, I recommend you seek professional help immediately.

SIGNS & SYMPTOMS

- Bleeding
- Drainage
- Infection
- Puncture Wound
- Swelling

TREATMENT

If you choose to treat your pet on your own or with the help of a veterinarian, here are some simple things you can do to help with the healing process.

1. First, clip the hair around the wound so hair is not covering the wound itself.

2. Wash the area with a mild shampoo and rinse completely.

You can use homeopathic Calendula tincture (4 drops per ounce of water) to rinse the area after you have cleaned it. You can repeat this process each day as needed to help the wound to heal with the minimum chance of secondary infection.

Animal Bites:

Cats: 5 drops each of **Black Currant, Black Poplar, European Walnut** twice per day for 7-10 days

Dogs: 5 drops each of **Black Currant, Black Poplar, European Walnut** twice per day for 7-10 days

Horses: 5 drops each of **Black Currant, Black Poplar, European Walnut** twice per day for 7-10 days

This will help with inflammation, collateral circulation healing and preventing infection. This should take no more than a week to 10 days to heal. If healing is not occurring within this time, seek veterinary help immediately. **NOTE: Black Poplar is a short-term remedy and should not be given more than 4 to 5 weeks.**

EAR INFECTIONS

Most ear infections are signs of chronic disease with secondary yeast and bacterial infections primarily considered to be the cause. They are secondary and will never clear up with drugs. Vaccines, chemicals, drugs, pesticides, herbicides, food, hereditary factors are part of this issue. You really need to work with an integrative veterinarian who understands management of chronic disease rather than a traditional veterinarian who follows a reductionism approach either with surgery, or with the use of suppressive drugs such as antibiotics, anti-fungal drugs, or steroids are used and drive the chronic condition even deeper into the animal.

It is imperative to keep the ear clean in order to make sure your animal is comfortable while you help him/her to detoxify and heal from the inside out. Use a mild ear wash, such as ALL EARS, by Wondercide (http://www.wondercide.com/ear-mite-treatment). All Ears is an all natural cedar-oil-based product that kills mites, their eggs and treats bacteria and yeast infections gently.

Warming the cleaning solution to body temperature is very important in the effectiveness of the cleaning and comfort of your pet. Just put the plastic bottle of ear wash in a half gallon of hot water and let it steep for 15 minutes. Take the warm solution and fill the ear, massage gently and let your pet shake out the wash. Repeat until the ears are clean. Do this as often as needed to keep the ear clean. By doing this, you are removing the media of wax on which the bacteria and yeast love to grow.

SIGNS & SYMPTOMS

- Ear Discharge
- Ears Swelling
- Itching
- Odor from Ears

TREATMENT

The main remedies for this condition are **Rowan Tree** and **Black Currant.** I recommend the following:

- **Rowan Tree and Black Currant**

    Cats: 1 to 3 drops of each, twice per day
    Dogs: 5 to 10 drops of each, twice per day

I recommend putting all animals on **Common Juniper** at the below dosage for a total of six weeks.

- **Common Juniper**

    Cats: 3 to 5 drops of **Common Juniper** once
             per day for a total of 6 weeks

    Dogs: 3 to 5 drops of **Common Juniper** once
             per day for a total of 6 weeks

After the six weeks is completed, take this same above dosage, 3 to 5 drops, once per week thereafter to detoxify and strengthen the liver and kidneys. Beginning each spring, repeat the six-week spring-cleaning protocol once again.

EAR MITES

These are most common in cats, but do occur in dogs as well. To make a correct diagnosis of this condition you need to have the waxy discharge from their ears examined under a microscope to find the actual parasite. Often times because they are discharging black wax it is assumed they have ear mites. Many times this is not the case but rather early symptoms of chronic disease. The main trigger for chronic ear discharge is vaccinations and chemicals. If your pet has ear issues, do not vaccinate them or use chemicals of any kind on them if at all possible.

Once the diagnosis of ear mites is made conclusively, you treat them with warm almond oil. Fill the ears with the warm oil outside and massage it into the ear for a minute, or as long as the animal will let you. The idea is to suffocate the mite since it mainly spends its entire life in the ear canal. Do this once every other day for a month to get all the hatching mites from the eggs that are in the ear canal.

SIGNS & SYMPTOMS

- Black Discharge from Ears
- Itching
- Shaking Head

TREATMENT

I recommend **Black Currant, Rowan Tree,** and **European Walnut** as the main Gemmotherapy remedies to treat ear mites.

- **Black Currant**

  Cats: 1 to 3 drops, one to four times per day
  Dogs: 5 to 10 drops, one to four times per day

I also put dogs on **Rowan Tree** and **European Walnut** to detoxify the body and help rid the ear of parasites and toxins. Continue this protocol until there is no further discharge or discomfort.

- **Rowan Tree** and **European Walnut**

  Dogs: 5 to 10 drops or each, once per day

FEAR OF NOISES

Fear of noises includes: thunder, gunshot, rushing water, or other sudden noises. Any pet who exhibits any of these fears should never be vaccinated or put on any drugs or chemicals which are neurotoxins. **Lime Tree, Common Birch** and **Common Juniper** are helpful in animals with this sensitivity.

SIGNS & SYMPTOMS

- Barks excessively when noises are heard
- Hides from sounds
- Startles easily when slight or loud noises are heard

TREATMENT

The main remedies for this condition are:

- **Common Birch and Lime Tree**

   Cats: 3 to 5 drops of each, one to four times per day, as needed for fear issues

   Dogs: 3 to 5 drops of each, one to four times per day, as needed for fear issues

I recommend putting all animals on **Common Juniper** at the below dosage for a total of six weeks.

- **Common Juniper**

    Cats: 3 to 5 drops of **Common Juniper** once per day for a total of 6 weeks

    Dogs: 3 to 5 drops of **Common Juniper** once per day for a total of 6 weeks

After the six-week regimen is completed, take this same above dosage, 3 to 5 drops, once per week thereafter to detoxify and strengthen the liver and kidneys.

Beginning each spring, repeat the six-week spring-cleaning protocol once again.

FOOD & GARBAGE POISONING

I recommend you fast your pet until all symptoms of poisoning have passed. In the meantime, make sure they have access to as much water as they want as long as they are not vomiting what they drink.

I also recommend supplementing their water with **100% New Zealand Colostrum** and let the pet drink as much as possible. **Fig Tree** and **Common Juniper** are the Gemmotherapy remedies to use to help detoxify and strengthen the gastro-intestinal system.

SIGNS & SYMPTOMS

- Abdominal pain
- Bloating
- Diarrhea
- Inappetence
- Nausea
- Vomiting

TREATMENT

- Give **100% New Zealand Bovine Colostrum,** by dissolving 500 mg of colostrum in four ounces of water. Let the pet drink as much as possible to help detoxify and strengthen the gastro-intestinal system.

- **Fig Tree**

  Cats: 3 to 5 drops, every hour until they are stable, then twice per day until they are eating normally.

  Dogs: 3 to 5 drops, every hour until they are stable, then twice per day until they are eating normally.

  I recommend putting all animals on **Common Juniper** at the above dosage for a total of six weeks.

- **Common Juniper**

  Cats: 3 to 5 drops of **Common Juniper** once per day for a total of 6 weeks

  Dogs: 3 to 5 drops of **Common Juniper** once per day for a total of 6 weeks

After the six-week-regimen is completed, take this same above dosage, 3 to 5 drops, once per week thereafter, to detoxify and strengthen the liver and kidneys. Beginning each spring, repeat the six-week spring-cleaning protocol once again.

FLY STRIKE

Prevention is always the best medicine. To prevent the flies from pestering your animals in the first place you want to make sure their immune systems are strong. To help them detoxify and build their immune systems, I suggest you apply Gemmotherapy remedies both topically and internally.

SIGNS & SYMPTOMS

- Bleeding
- Crust
- Itching
- Loss of Hair on Ear Tips

TREATMENT

Topically I recommend a few drops of **European Walnut** to prevent fly strike and homeopathic **Calendula cream** on the ears as needed for healing.

Internally I recommend **European Walnut** and **Rye Grain** to help repel the flies.

- **European Walnut** and **Rye Grain**

  Dogs: 5 to 10 drops twice per day as long as needed to help repel the flies

Horses: 5 to 10 drops twice per day as long as needed to help repel the flies

I recommend putting all animals on **Common Juniper** at the below dosage for a total of six weeks.

- **Common Juniper**

    Cats: 3 to 5 drops of **Common Juniper** once per day for a total of 6 weeks

    Dogs: 3 to 5 drops of **Common Juniper** once per day for a total of 6 weeks

    Horses: 3 to 5 drops of **Common Juniper** once per day for a total of 6 weeks

After the six-week-regimen is completed, take this same above dosage, 3 to 5 drops, once per week thereafter to detoxify and strengthen the liver and kidneys.

Beginning each spring, repeat the six-week spring-cleaning protocol once again.

FOXTAILS & FOREIGN BODIES

This is more of an issue in dogs and cats, not horses. If a dog has been in a field with foxtails and starts shaking its head violently and scratching at its ear, it probably has a foxtail down in its ear and is in pain. You can fill the ear with almond oil and gently massage it around until the dog is more comfortable. I would recommend doing this outside because he is going to shake his head and oil is bound to decorate everything within reach of his shake.

The point of this exercise is to soften the foxtail so it won't do any immediate harm to the animal, and further, in hopes that the foxtail will fly out with the shaking of his head. You can repeat this multiple times until he is comfortable. This usually will allow you time to wait until your regular veterinarian's office is open and help you to stay out of the veterinary emergency room, saving your pet and you fear and discomfort, and lots of money too!

SIGNS & SYMPTOMS

- Excessive Licking and Scratching
- Opening in Skin with Drainage
- Shaking of Head or Sneezing
- Swelling

TREATMENT

The main remedies for this condition are **Rowan Tree** and **Black Currant.** I recommend the following:

- **Rowan Tree and Black Currant**

  Cats: 1 to 3 drops of each, twice per day
  Dogs: 5 to 10 drops of each, twice per day

GINGIVITIS & MOUTH INFLAMMATION

Gingivitis is a symptom of chronic disease and should be managed as such. Infections are secondary and require the help of a veterinarian to determine the need for surgery and antibiotics.

I recommend dogs and cats chew on raw bones. Beef ribs for dogs and chicken wings for cats. I suggest you limit the amount of time for chewing the bones to 15 minutes per day until they get the cleaning effect of the bones and then as needed to help keep their teeth and gums healthier.

SIGNS & SYMPTOMS

- Odor
- Redness of Gums
- Swelling of Gums

TREATMENT

- **Rowan Tree and European Walnut**

    Cats: 1 to 3 drops of each, twice per day until healed

    Dogs: 5 to 10 drops of each, twice per day until healed

    Horses: 5 to 10 drops of each, twice per day until healed

- **Common Juniper**

  Cats: 3 to 5 drops of **Common Juniper** once
  per day for a total of 6 weeks

  Dogs: 3 to 5 drops of **Common Juniper** once
  per day for a total of 6 weeks

  Horses: 3 to 5 drops of **Common Juniper** once
  per day for a total of 6 weeks

I recommend putting all animals on **Common Juniper** at the above dosage for a total of six weeks.

After the six weeks is completed, take this same above dosage, 3 to 5 drops, once per week thereafter to detoxify and strengthen the liver and kidneys.

Beginning each spring, repeat the six-week spring-cleaning protocol once again.

HEART DISEASE

I've seen this condition mostly in cats and dogs. You should never vaccinate or put them on any drugs or chemicals which are neurotoxins. Make sure you are providing **100% New Zealand Bovine Colostrum** daily to help strengthen the heart, gastro-intestinal tract and immune system.

SIGNS & SYMPTOMS

- Congestion of Lungs
- Coughing with Exertion or During Sleep
- Difficulty Breathing with or without Exertion
- Fainting

TREATMENT

- Give **100% New Zealand Bovine Colostrum** at a dose of 500 mg per 25 pounds of body weight, twice per day.

- **Black Currant, English Hawthorn, European Alder, European Olive**

  Cats: 3 to 5 drops of each, twice per day
  Dogs: 3 to 5 drops of each, twice per day

- **Common Juniper**

    Cats: 3 to 5 drops of **Common Juniper** once
            per day for a total of 6 weeks

    Dogs: 3 to 5 drops of **Common Juniper** once
            per day for a total of 6 weeks

I recommend putting all animals on **Common Juniper** at the above dosage for a total of six weeks.

After the six weeks is completed, take this same above dosage, 3 to 5 drops, once per week thereafter to detoxify and strengthen the liver and kidneys.

Beginning each spring, repeat the six-week spring-cleaning protocol once again.

HIP DYSPLASIA

This is a common diagnosis seen mainly in dogs. I recommend you dose with **Wild Woodvine** and **Common Birch** until they have no more symptoms and then weekly or as needed thereafter for detoxifying and strengthening the joints.

SIGNS & SYMPTOMS

- Difficulty Rising
- Gait Swelling
- Malformation of Hips
- Painful Stiff Rear
- Knees Held Close Together When Sitting to Relieve Discomfort
- Knees Held Close Together When Standing/Walking Due to Painful Hip Joints

TREATMENT

- **Common Birch** and **Wild Woodvine**

  Dogs: 5 to 10 drops of each, twice a day until there are no symptoms and then weekly or as needed thereafter for detoxifying and strengthening the joints.

I recommend putting all animals on **Common Juniper** at the below dosage for a total of six weeks.

- **Common Juniper**

    Dogs: 3 to 5 drops of **Common Juniper** once per day for a total of 6 weeks

    After the six-week regimen is completed, take this same above dosage, 3 to 5 drops, once per week thereafter to detoxify and strengthen the liver and kidneys.

    Beginning each spring, repeat the six-week spring-cleaning protocol once again.

HOT SPOTS

A common situation faced by many pet owners is that of acute inflammatory situations. This could be caused by an insect bite from a flea, fly, or tick; or from a contact allergy from an irritating substance, such as chemicals, pollen, or toxins of any kind. I have seen hundreds, if not thousands, of allergic-reaction cases and found the following course of action to be very helpful in relieving the discomfort pets may be experiencing.

Dogs will often show allergic reactions through their skin in the form of hot spots, rashes or itching. **Black Currant** is excellent for all of these symptoms and can be dosed as below, depending upon the need of the patient.

SIGNS & SYMPTOMS

- Biting and Scratching until Skin is irritated
- Dry or Wet Appearance
- Itching
- Loss Of Hair
- Swelling

TREATMENT

If the animal has gotten into something toxic or irritating, your first concern is to bathe the animal with a mild shampoo. Before you bathe the animal, you can give him/her the following:

- **Black Currant**

  Cats: 4 to 10 drops every 15 minutes until the patient is more comfortable and then as needed thereafter.

  Dogs: 4 to 10 drops every 15 minutes until the patient is more comfortable and then as needed thereafter.

  Horses: 4 to 10 drops every 15 minutes until the patient is more comfortable and then as needed thereafter.

- Topically, mix 1 drop of **Black Currant** per ounce of water and apply to areas of swelling or itching to help reduce the inflammation causing the irritation.

As I have mentioned in other parts of this book, these tinctures can be applied transdermally and can be used on any surface of the body except for the eyes. You can rub them around the perimeter of the eyes but do not get them into the eyes due to the potential irritation they may cause the animals. If you should get some into their eyes, wash them out thoroughly with water until the animal is comfortable.

- **Common Juniper**

    Cats: 3 to 5 drops of **Common Juniper** once per day for a total of 6 weeks

    Dogs: 3 to 5 drops of **Common Juniper** once per day for a total of 6 weeks

    Horses: 3 to 5 drops of **Common Juniper** once per day for a total of 6 weeks

    I recommend putting all animals on **Common Juniper** at the above dosage for a total of six weeks.

    After the six-week-regimen is completed, take this same above dosage, 3 to 5 drops, once per week thereafter to detoxify and strengthen the liver and kidneys.

    Beginning each spring, repeat the six-week spring-cleaning protocol once again.

HYPOPYON (EYE PROBLEMS)

Pus behind the cornea known as hypopyon can occur in cats and dogs. With a condition such as this I recommend you see a veterinarian immediately.

SIGNS & SYMPTOMS

- Discoloration of The Interior of The Eye Chamber
- Pus in the Interior Chamber Of The Eye

TREATMENT

Until the eye is healed, I recommend the following:

- **Black Currant, Common Birch** and **Hedge Maple**

  Cats: 3 to 5 drops of each, twice a day until the eye is healed

  Dogs: 3 to 5 drops of each, twice a day until the eye is healed

- **Common Juniper**

  Cats: 3 to 5 drops of **Common Juniper** once per day for a total of 6 weeks

  Dogs: 3 to 5 drops of **Common Juniper** once per day for a total of 6 weeks

I recommend putting all animals on **Common Juniper** at the above dosage for a total of six weeks.

After the six-week-regimen is completed, take this same above dosage, 3 to 5 drops, once per week thereafter to detoxify and strengthen the liver and kidneys.

Beginning each spring, repeat the six-week spring-cleaning protocol once again.

INFECTIONS

The most common infections we see in animals involve the skin, ears, eyes, lungs, bladder, kidneys, liver, pancreas, central nervous system, blood (systemic) and lymphatic system. The reason for these infections is due to a less-than-optimal state of health of the animal. The bacterial, viral and fungal infective agents are very common in their bodies and the environment. When the body is in a state of homeostasis, it lives in a symbiotic relationship with these microorganisms. When the body is in a weakened state, secondary to physical and or emotional stresses, it is susceptible to excessive proliferation of these organisms, resulting in a secondary infection.

SIGNS & SYMPTOMS

- Elevated Temperature
- Elevated White Blood Count
- Fever
- Inflammation

TREATMENT

- **European Walnut** and **Hedge Maple**

  Cats: 3 to 5 drops of each, twice per day
  Dogs: 3 to 5 drops of each, twice per day
  Horses: 3 to 5 drops of each, twice per day

INTERVERTEBRAL DISC DISEASE (Slipped Disc)

This is most often seen in dogs but does occur in cats as well. The forming of bone spurs along the ventral aspect of the spinal column is a result of chronic inflammation and instability of the spine.

SIGNS & SYMPTOMS

- Pain
- Paralysis of Rear Legs
- Sudden Onset
- Weakness

TREATMENT

- **Black Currant, Common Birch** and **Mountain Pine**

  Cats: 3 to 5 drops of each, twice per day
  Dogs: 3 to 5 drops of each, twice per day

  I recommend putting all animals on **Common Juniper** at the above dosage for a total of six weeks.

- **Common Juniper**

  Cats: 3 to 5 drops of **Common Juniper** once
           per day for a total of 6 weeks

  Dogs: 3 to 5 drops of **Common Juniper** once
           per day for a total of 6 weeks

  After the six-week-regimen is completed, take this
  same above dosage, 3 to 5 drops, once per week
  thereafter to detoxify and strengthen the liver and
  kidneys.

ITCHING

Expose a dog to a substance to which he is sensitive, and you can just about bet that the outer symptom will be an itch that drives him crazy. This could be caused by contact with chemicals, plant materials, food allergies, vaccinations and drugs. Your first step is to eliminate the causative agent if at all possible and bathe as needed to remove the substance with which they came into contact topically. Itching can many times be a sign of chronic disease in your pet and needs to be evaluated as such. This is a time when you need to have an integrative veterinarian who understands the energetics of healing.

One of the most common triggers for itching in dogs and cats is vaccinations. I highly recommend only core puppy or kitten vaccinations be allowed, and **NO** boosters. I would not recommend any vaccines if the cat or dog is showing any signs of allergic tendencies.

SIGNS & SYMPTOMS

- Excessive Licking or Scratching

TREATMENT

The main remedy I use for itching in the dog, cat or horse is **Black Currant.** Your first concern is to bathe

the animal if it has something toxic or irritating on it, using a mild, lavender-based shampoo. Before you bathe the animal, you can give him/her **Black Currant** at the following dosage:

- **Black Currant**

  Cats: 5 to 10 drops every 15 minutes until the patient is more comfortable and then as needed thereafter.

  Dogs: 5 to 10 drops every 15 minutes until the patient is more comfortable and then as needed thereafter.

  Horses: 5 to 10 drops every 15 minutes until the patient is more comfortable and then as needed thereafter.

As I have mentioned in other parts of this book, these tinctures can be applied transdermally, and can be used on any surface of the body except for the eyes. You can rub them around the perimeter of the eyes but do not get them into the eyes due to the potential irritation they may cause the animals. If you should get some into their eyes, wash them out thoroughly with water until the animal is comfortable.

- Topically, mix 1 drop of **Black Currant** per ounce of water and apply to areas of swelling or itching to help reduce the inflammation causing the irritation.

If the issue of itching is of a chronic nature (lasting over periods of months or years), I recommend using **Cedar of Lebanon** along with the **Black Currant**.

- **Cedar of Lebanon** and **Black Currant**

  Cats: 1 to 3 drops of each, twice per day
  Dogs: 5 to 10 drops of each, twice per day
  Horses: 5 to 10 drops of each, twice per day

I recommend putting all animals on **Common Juniper** at the below dosage for a total of six weeks.

- **Common Juniper**

  Cats: 3 to 5 drops of **Common Juniper** once per day for a total of 6 weeks
  Dogs: 3 to 5 drops of **Common Juniper** once per day for a total of 6 weeks
  Horses: 3 to 5 drops of **Common Juniper** once per day for a total of 6 weeks

After the six-week-regimen is completed, take this same above dosage, 3 to 5 drops, once per week thereafter, to detoxify and strengthen the liver and kidneys.

Beginning each spring, repeat the six-week spring-cleaning protocol once again.

KIDNEY FAILURE

This is very common system failure in both cats and dogs. Vaccines, drugs and chemicals can cause or trigger this condition. I recommend you seek veterinary care immediately if your pet is showing signs of kidney failure. You should have blood work and urinalysis done immediately to determine if this is the case or not.

SIGNS & SYMPTOMS

- Increased Thirst
- Increased Urination
- Loss Of Appetite
- Loss Of Weight
- Odor From Mouth
- Vomiting
- Lethargy
- Weakness

TREATMENT

- **Black Currant, Common Birch** and **Silver Birch**

  Cats: 3 to 5 drops of each, twice a day
  Dogs: 3 to 5 drops of each, twice a day

I recommend fresh filtered water and or heated fluids subcutaneously if the cat or dog is not drinking enough to stay hydrated.

I also recommend putting all animals on **Common Juniper** at the below dosage for a total of six weeks.

- **Common Juniper**

  Cats: 3 to 5 drops of **Common Juniper** once per day for a total of 6 weeks
  Dogs: 3 to 5 drops of **Common Juniper** once per day for a total of 6 weeks

After the six-week-regimen is completed, take this same above dosage, 3 to 5 drops, once per week thereafter, to detoxify and strengthen the liver and kidneys.

Beginning each spring, repeat the six-week spring-cleaning protocol once again.

LIVER DISORDER

This condition affects cats and dogs. You should never vaccinate or put them on any drugs or chemicals which are neurotoxins. Make sure you are providing **100% New Zealand Bovine Colostrum** to help strengthen the liver. **Black Currant, Common Birch, Common Juniper** and **Rosemary** should be given until the patient's liver function is returned to normal, then dose weekly for maintenance and prevention.

SIGNS & SYMPTOMS

- Inappetence
- Increased Thirst And Urination
- Nausea
- Possible Jaundice
- Vomiting of Bile
- Weight Loss

TREATMENT

- Give **100% New Zealand Bovine Colostrum** at a dose of 500 mg per 25 pounds of body weight, twice per day.

- **Black Currant, Common Birch,** and **Rosemary**

  Cats: 3 to 5 drops of each, twice per day
  Dogs: 3 to 5 drops of each, twice per day

- **Common Juniper**

  Cats: 3 to 5 drops of **Common Juniper** once per day for a total of 6 weeks

  Dogs: 3 to 5 drops of **Common Juniper** once per day for a total of 6 weeks

I recommend putting all animals on **Common Juniper** at the above dosage for a total of six weeks.

After the six-week-regimen is completed, take this same above dosage, 3 to 5 drops, once per week thereafter, to detoxify and strengthen the liver and kidneys.

Beginning each spring, repeat the six-week spring-cleaning protocol once again.

MANGE

There are mainly two forms of mange we usually see in dogs, **Sarcoptic** (contagious) and **Demodectic** (non-contagious). Sarcoptic is very itchy and can be picked up by humans and other animals. You'll need to use other methods of treatment to contain the mites but you can use the following Gemmotherapy remedies to aid in the process of healing.

In both forms of mange I recommend **Black Currant** for itching and adrenal support, **European Walnut** for helping with infections and making the animals more resistant to the parasites, and **Rye Grain** to detoxify the skin and help with the healing process of the skin.

SIGNS & SYMPTOMS

- Eruptions around Hair Follicles
- Itching
- Loss of Hair (Localized or Generalized)

TREATMENT

- **Black Currant, European Walnut,** and **Rye Grain**

  Dogs: 5 to 10 drops once per day until animal is free of any mange symptoms.

- **Common Juniper**

  Dogs: 3 to 5 drops of **Common Juniper** once per day for a total of 6 weeks

  After the six-week-regimen is completed, take this same above dosage, 3 to 5 drops, once per week thereafter, to detoxify and strengthen the liver and kidneys.

  Beginning each spring, repeat the six-week spring-cleaning protocol once again.

NOSEBLEED

Nosebleeds are often caused by foxtails. If you see a dog start sneezing after walking in an area with foxtails (thistles), consider that a foxtail has possibly been inhaled into the nasal cavity. I find that if you put 5 to 10 drops of almond oil into the nose it will help him sneeze it out or prevent it from going deeper into the nose. You should seek veterinary help if the sneezing persists.

SIGNS & SYMPTOMS

- Bleeding from nose
- Sneezing

TREATMENT

- **Briar Rose**

    Dogs: 5 to 10 drops every 15 minutes until the sneezing stops

If you do not see improvement in the sneezing within a half hour, seek veterinary attention.

OVERHEATING

This is more a condition seen in dogs and horses due to extreme heat with exertion. The obvious thing to do is be mindful of the temperatures when working your dog or horse. Make sure you let them cool down often and have plenty of water at all times and shade whenever possible.

If they do become overheated, placing cold packs around the head, ears and neck will help them to cool their blood more quickly.

SIGNS & SYMPTOMS

- Elevated Temperature
- Lethargy
- Panting
- Prostration

TREATMENT

I would start them on **Black Currant** and **Common Birch** and **Lime Tree.** Do this until they are breathing normally and comfortably. You might consider not exercising your pet further if the conditions will cause him to overheat again the same day.

- **Black Currant, Common Birch, and Lime Tree**

    Dogs: 5 to 10 drops every 5 minutes, until
                  comfortable again

    Horses: 5 to 10 drops every 5 minutes, until
                  comfortable again

POSTPARTUM CONDITIONS

I recommend **100% New Zealand Bovine Colostrum** even before breeding the animal, until the newborns are weaned. Once the cat or dog goes into labor, I recommend they be put on **Raspberry** and **Black Currant.**

SIGNS & SYMPTOMS

- Abnormal discharge from vulva
- Cramping
- Excessive neediness
- Excessive restlessness
- Irritability
- Lack of milk for puppies or kittens
- Lack of nursing skills
- Refusing puppies or kittens
- Retained placenta or fetus

TREATMENT

- Give **100% New Zealand Bovine Colostrum** at a dose of 500 mg per 25 pounds of body weight, once per day prior to breeding, until the newborns are weaned.

- Once the last birthing is complete, continue **100% New Zealand Bovine Colostrum** twice per day until there is no longer any discharge from the vagina.

Once the cat or dog goes into labor, I recommend the following:

- **Raspberry** and **Black Currant**

Cats: 3 to 5 drops every hour during labor
Dogs: 3 to 5 drops every hour during labor

PROSTATE AFFECTIONS

This is a condition of dogs. I recommend never vaccinate, nor use flea, tick, chemicals or heartworm medication on animals with prostate issues. I recommend **Black Currant, Rosemary** and **Common Birch** until the prostate gland is back to normal size with no clinical symptoms. After that, I recommend weekly dosing.

SIGNS & SYMPTOMS

- Blood In Urine
- Frequent Attempt To Urinate With Little Urine
- Painful Urination
- Small Amounts Of Urine Multiple Times Per Day
- Straining With No Urine Release

TREATMENT

- **Black Currant, Common Birch** and **Rosemary**

  Dogs: 5 to 10 drops of each, twice per day until the prostate gland is back to normal size with no clinical symptoms.

After that I recommend 5 to 10 drops of each, one time, weekly.

- **Common Juniper**

  Cats: 3 to 5 drops of **Common Juniper** once per day for a total of 6 weeks
  Dogs: 3 to 5 drops of **Common Juniper** once per day for a total of 6 weeks
  Horses: 3 to 5 drops of **Common Juniper** once per day for a total of 6 weeks

I recommend putting all animals on **Common Juniper** at the above dosage for a total of six weeks.

After the six-week-regimen is completed, take this same above dosage, 3 to 5 drops, once per week thereafter, to detoxify and strengthen the liver and kidneys.

Beginning each spring, repeat the six-week spring-cleaning protocol once again.

RANULA

This is a rare condition mainly seen in dogs. In my opinion, the main trigger of ranula in dogs is vaccinations. For this reason I recommend you never re-vaccinate a dog if they develop this condition.

Use **Rowan Tree** since it is the main draining remedy for the ears, nose, throat, head, and neck areas of the body and **European Walnut** for infections.

SIGNS & SYMPTOMS

- Swelling under Tongue
- Soft Fluid-Filled Mass

TREATMENT

- **European Walnut** and **Rowan Tree**

    Dogs: 5 to 10 drops of each, twice per day until the gums are healed.

- **Common Juniper**

    Dogs: 3 to 5 drops of **Common Juniper** once per day for a total of 6 weeks

After the six-week-regimen is completed, take this same above dosage, 3 to 5 drops, once per week thereafter to detoxify and strengthen the liver and kidneys.

Beginning each spring, repeat the six-week spring-cleaning protocol once again.

RETAINED TESTICLE (CRYPTORCHIDISM)

This is a condition mainly seen in dogs. Vaccines can trigger this condition and for that reason I recommend not vaccinating dogs until they are 12 weeks of age, or not at all.

If you vaccinate at 12-weeks, only give Parvo vaccine by itself and wait two weeks, then give distemper. No other vaccines should be given at this time and never give any vaccines at the same time you have to vaccinate for rabies.

SIGNS & SYMPTOMS

- Absence of One or Both Testicles in Scrotum

TREATMENT

- **Common Birch** and **European Oak**

  Dogs: 3 to 5 drops, twice per day. Repeat daily until the testicle descends.

RINGWORM

This is a fungal infection more common in cats but does occur in horses and dogs as well. **Rye Grain**, **Prim Wort** and **English Elm** are the three main remedies I recommend for helping the animal heal.

This is a potentially contagious infection to other animals and people. Consult your veterinarian for professional care on handling this issue within your home and around other animals.

SIGNS & SYMPTOMS

- Circular Losses of Hair
- Crusts
- Itching
- Swelling

- **English Elm, Prim Wort,** and **Rye Grain**

    Cats: 1 to 3 drops of each, twice per day until
    healed

    Dogs: 5 to 10 drops of each, twice per day until
    healed

    Horses: 5 to 10 drops of each, twice per day until
    healed

SKIN INFECTIONS & ERUPTIONS

All skin eruptions are usually an outward symptom caused by internal issues discharging through the skin or a result of contact from something in the environment, such as external parasites, irritants, chemicals, plant material, etc. First thing to do is clean the skin with a gentle shampoo. Giving the animal a second shampooing depends on the odor and whether the dog, horse or cat feels dirty to the touch.

Most animals with eruptions or infections for the first time, with no history of chronic skin issues, will respond well to using **Black Currant, European Walnut** and **Rye Grain.**

SIGNS & SYMPTOMS

- Itching
- Odor
- Oozing
- Painful to Touch
- Redness
- Scabs
- Swelling

TREATMENT

If the animal has gotten into something toxic or irritating, your first concern is to bathe the animal with a mild shampoo. Before you bathe the animal, you can give him/her the following:

- **Black Currant**

    Cats:　　1 to 3 drops every 15 minutes until the patient is more comfortable and then as needed thereafter.

    Dogs:　　4 to 10 drops every 15 minutes until the patient is more comfortable and then as needed thereafter.

    Horses:　4 to 10 drops every 15 minutes until the patient is more comfortable and then as needed thereafter.

Once the animal is comfortable, usually after 1 to 4 repeated treatments, I go to a maintenance dose of **Black Currant, European Walnut** and **Rye Grain** in the following amounts:

- **Black Currant**

  Cats: 1 to 3 drops twice per day until the skin is healed

  Dogs: 5 to 10 drops twice per day until the skin is healed

  Horses: 5 to 10 drops twice per day until the skin is healed

- **European Walnut** and **Rye Grain**

  Cats: 1 to 3 drops once per day until the skin is healed

  Dogs: 5 to 10 drops once per day until the skin is healed

  Horses: 5 to 10 drops once per day until the skin is healed

As I have mentioned in other parts of this book, these tinctures can be applied transdermally, and can be used on any surface of the body except for the eyes. You can rub them around the perimeter of the eyes but do not get them into the eyes due to the potential irritation they may cause the animals. If you should get some into their eyes, wash them out thoroughly with water until the animal is comfortable.

- Topically, mix 1 drop of **Black Currant** and 1 drop of **European Walnut** each, per ounce of water and apply to areas of swelling or itching to help reduce the inflammation causing the irritation.

I also recommend putting all animals on **Common Juniper** at the below dosage for a total of six weeks.

- **Common Juniper**

Cats:　3 to 5 drops,once per day for a total of 6 weeks
Dogs:　3 to 5 drops,once per day for a total of 6 weeks
Horses: 3 to 5 drops,once per day for a total of 6 weeks

After completing the six-week-regimen, take this same above dosage, 3 to 5 drops, once per week thereafter to detoxify and strengthen the liver and kidneys. Beginning each spring, repeat the six-week spring-cleaning protocol once again.

SNAKE BITES

Snake bites are very dangerous and warrant immediate attention at a veterinary hospital. Here are some things you can do to help with the healing process. I recommend **Purification Blend** of essential oils be applied directly on the bite and repeated every 15 minutes until there is no pain. Once the pain stops, repeat only as needed or twice per day until completely healed. The link to this oil can be found on my website: http://thepetwhisperer.com/essential_oil.html

SIGNS & SYMPTOMS

- Bleeding
- Bruising
- Lethargy
- Painful
- Puncture Wounds

TREATMENT

- **Black Currant, Black Poplar, European Walnut**

    Cats: 5 drops of each, twice per day for 7-10 days

    Dogs: 5 drops of each, twice per day for 7-10 days

    Horses: 5 drops of each, twice per day for 7-10 days

This will help with inflammation, collateral circulation healing and preventing infection. This should take no more than a week to 10 days to heal. If healing is not occurring within this time, seek veterinary help immediately. **NOTE: Black Poplar is a short-term remedy and should not be given more than 4 to 5 weeks.**

SNEEZING & NASAL CONGESTION

Sneezing and congestion are usually due to inflammatory states, secondary to built-up toxins in the tissue of the nasal cavities, resulting in nasal discharge and sneezing.

Oftentimes you will see this happen after a vaccination or application of a chemical topically or orally. The next most common situation would be secondary infections from bacteria, viruses or fungal infections. The infections are secondary to the toxicity that weakens this area of the body and allows the abnormal proliferation of these microorganisms.

SIGNS & SYMPTOMS

- Discharge from Nostrils
- Episodes of Sneezing
- Labored Breathing
- Nasal Sounds when Breathing.
- Rapid Involuntary

TREATMENT

The main remedies for this condition are **Rowan Tree** and **Black Currant.** I recommend the following:

- **Rowan Tree and Black Currant**

  Cats: 1 to 3 drops of each, twice per day
  Dogs: 5 to 10 drops of each, twice per day

If the sneezing and nasal congestion are cause by an allergy, you can start the animal on:

- **Briar Rose and Black Currant**

  Cats: 1 to 3 drops of each, every 15 minutes until you see improvement, stop and repeat as needed.

  Dogs: 5 to 10 drops of each, every 15 minutes until you see improvement, stop and repeat as needed.

Nasal issue triggers are commonly those of over vaccinating and toxic chemicals with which the animal comes into contact.

SPONDYLITIS

This is most often seen in dogs but does occur in cats as well. The forming of bone spurs along the ventral aspect of the spinal column is a result of chronic inflammation and instability of the spine. I recommend it be treated daily with **Mountain Pine, Black Currant and Common Birch.** Once there are no further symptoms, I dose weekly thereafter to help detoxify and strengthen the spine.

SIGNS & SYMPTOMS

- Calcification of Spinal Vertebrae
- Difficult Rising or Sitting
- Difficulty Jumping Up
- Painful, Stiff Back

TREATMENT

- **Black Currant, Common Birch, Mountain Pine**

  Cats: 3 to 5 drops of each, twice per day
  Dogs: 3 to 5 drops of each, twice per day

Once there are no further symptoms, I dose 3 to 5 drops, once a week thereafter to help detoxify and strengthen the spine.

I also recommend putting all animals on **Common Juniper** at the below dosage for a total of six weeks.

- **Common Juniper**

  Cats: 3 to 5 drops of **Common Juniper** once
             per day for a total of 6 weeks

  Dogs: 3 to 5 drops of **Common Juniper** once
             per day for a total of 6 weeks

After completing the six weeks, take this same above dosage, 3 to 5 drops, once per week thereafter to detoxify and strengthen the liver and kidneys.

Beginning each spring, repeat the six-week spring-cleaning protocol once again.

SPRAINS & STRAINS

This is a common occurrence more in dogs than cats. The treatment is the same for both species. I recommend you dose with **Wild Woodvine, European Grapevine, Common Juniper** and **Common Birch.**

SIGNS & SYMPTOMS

- Lameness
- Pain
- Stiffness
- Swelling

TREATMENT

- **Grapevine, Common Birch** and **Wild Woodvine**

Cats: 3 to 5 drops of all three twice per day
Dogs: 3 to 5 drops of all three twice per day

Treat them daily until they have no symptoms and then weekly or as needed thereafter for detoxifying and strengthen the joints.

I also recommend putting all animals on **Common Juniper** at the below dosage for a total of six weeks.

146

Common Juniper

Cats: 3 to 5 drops of **Common Juniper** once per day for a total of 6 weeks

Dogs: 3 to 5 drops of **Common Juniper** once per day for a total of 6 weeks

After completing the six weeks, take this same above dosage, 3 to 5 drops, once per week thereafter to detoxify and strengthen the liver and kidneys.

Beginning each spring, repeat the six-week spring-cleaning protocol once again.

THYROID DISEASE (Hyperthyroidism)

One of the main triggers for this condition is vaccines causing an autoimmune condition of the thyroid gland. This can be either in the form of Hyperthyroidism (overactive, mainly in the cat) or Hypothyroid (underactive, mainly in the dog). I recommend you never vaccinate, use chemicals or drugs of any kind in animals with any form of thyroid dysfunction.

Make sure you are providing **100% New Zealand Bovine Colostrum** to help strengthen the liver, heart, gastro-intestinal tract, and the immune system.

SIGNS & SYMPTOMS

- Elevated Blood Pressure
- Excessive Appetite With Weight Loss
- Rapid Heart Beat
- Vomiting

TREATMENT

- Give **100% New Zealand Bovine Colostrum** at a dose of 500 mg. per 25 pounds of body weight, twice per day.

- **Bloodtwig Dogberry**

  Cats: 3 to 5 drops twice per day
  Dogs: 3 to 5 drops twice per day

  I continue this until all thyroid values are normal and then weekly thereafter for protection.

  I also recommend putting all animals on **Common Juniper** at the below dosage for a total of six weeks.

  Common Juniper

  Cats: 3 to 5 drops of **Common Juniper** once per day for a total of 6 weeks
  Dogs: 3 to 5 drops of **Common Juniper** once per day for a total of 6 weeks

After completing the six weeks, take this same above dosage, 3 to 5 drops, once per week thereafter to detoxify and strengthen the liver and kidneys. Beginning each spring, repeat the six-week spring-cleaning protocol once again.

THYROID DISEASE (Hypothyroidism)

One of the main triggers for this condition is overuse of vaccines, causing an autoimmune condition of the thyroid gland. This can be either in the form of Hyperthyroidism (overactive, mainly in the cat) or Hypothyroid (underactive, mainly in the dog). I recommend you never vaccinate, use chemicals or drugs of any kind in animals with any form of thyroid dysfunction.

Make sure you are providing **100% New Zealand Bovine Colostrum** to help strengthen the liver, heart, gastro-intestinal tract, and the immune system.

SIGNS & SYMPTOMS

- Constipation
- Dry Coat
- Excessive Appetite
- Hair Loss
- Lack Of Endurance
- Weight Gain

TREATMENT

- Give **100% New Zealand Bovine Colostrum** at a dose of 500 mg. per 25 pounds of body weight, twice per day.

- **Bloodtwig Dogberry**

  Cats: 3 to 5 drops twice per day
  Dogs: 3 to 5 drops twice per day

  I continue this until all thyroid values are normal and then weekly thereafter for protection.

  I also recommend putting all animals on **Common Juniper** at the below dosage for a total of six weeks.

  Common Juniper
  Cats: 3 to 5 drops of **Common Juniper** once per day for a total of 6 weeks
  Dogs: 3 to 5 drops of **Common Juniper** once per day for a total of 6 weeks

After the six-week-regimen is completed, take this same above dosage, 3 to 5 drops, once per week thereafter to detoxify and strengthen the liver and kidneys.

URINARY INCONTINENCE

This is a common issue in dogs. Approximately twenty-five percent or more of spayed females will have issues of urinary incontinence. I recommend you try not to spay your dog until she has had at least one heat or more. This will allow her to develop hormonally before removing her uterus and ovaries.

The main remedies I use for female dogs are **Giant Redwood** and **Wine Berry** as needed for leakage of urine. The **Giant Redwood** is to help with bladder sphincter tone and **Wine Berry** is to help balance female hormones.

The main remedies I use in male dogs are **Giant Redwood** and **European Oak** as needed for leakage of urine. **Giant Redwood** helps with bladder sphincter tone and **European Oak** helps balance male hormones.

SIGNS & SYMPTOMS

- Involuntary Urination
- Leakage of Urine while Resting or Sleeping

TREATMENT

- **Giant Redwood** and **Wine Berry**

  Female Dogs: 5 to 10 drops, twice per day or as needed for leakage of urine

- **Giant Redwood** and **European Oak**

  Male Dogs: 5 to 10 drops, twice per day or as needed for leakage of urine

VOMITING

Vomiting is the body's way of discharging toxic materials from the stomach. If the animal is in pain and distress, or vomiting blood, seek immediate veterinary care.

The goal of our treatment is to help the animal detoxify as quickly as possible and make sure it is hydrated. The first thing you want to verify is that the animal has not gotten into anything toxic or eaten something that could cause obstructive disease. If either of these is the case, seek immediate veterinary help.

Immediately cease giving your pet any food until he or she is stable. Always provide liquids unless the animal is vomiting water when it drinks it and cannot keep it down. If this is the case, seek your local veterinarian for assistance.

SIGNS & SYMPTOMS

- Inappetence
- Lethargy
- Nausea

TREATMENT

If the animal can hold water down, I recommend starting the pet on **Fig Tree** and **European Grape Vine**. Repeat the dosage below each time the animal vomits. Wait a few minutes after they vomit to let their stomachs settle and then repeat the dose. As long as the vomiting decreases and is less and less frequent, your pet will be fine. If this is not the case, it's time to seek professional help.

- **Fig Tree** and **European Walnut**

  Cats: 1 to 3 drops of each
  Dogs: 5 to 10 drops of each
  Horse: 5 to 10 drops of each

DRAINING & DETOXIFICATION

There are several main organs known as emunctories, which are responsible for detoxifying the body and helping eliminate cellular waste such as toxins, poisons, chemicals and heavy metals. It is important that these main organs are cleared out before proceeding with the restorative therapy. The chart below outlines the best remedies to use to improve the function of each of those organs. Based on the individualized sensitivity of the animal, it is recommended that you give between 1-5 drops several times a day.

	Black Poplar	Bloodtwig Dogberry	Briar Rose	Cedar of Lebanon	Common Birch	Common Juniper	European Alder	Fig Tree	Lime Tree	Lithy Tree	Rowan Tree	Rosemary	Wine Berry
Artery Drainer	X	X											
Bladder Drainer													X
Dermal Drainer				X									
Endocrine Drainer		X											
Galbladder Drainer												X	
Heart Drainer		X											
Intestinal Drainer								X					
Kidney Drainer				X	X	X							
Lung Drainer										X			
Nerve Drainer								X	X				
Sinus Drainer			X										
Stomach Drainer							X	X					
Thyroid Drainer		X											
Universal Drainer				X									
Venous Drainer				X							X		

Imagination is more important than knowledge!

Albert Einstein

Gemmotherapy Remedies

(Common Name)

Black Currant (Ribes nigrum)

- Adrenal failure
- Adrenal imbalance-strengthens the adrenal glands
- Allergic conditions
- Anaphylaxis
- Asthma
- Balances the animal's immune system
- Bites and Stings
- Blood Urea Nitrogen
- Conjunctivitis
- Corneal disease
- Corticosteroid alternative
- Ear, Nose and Throat
- Fleas
- Heartworm
- Helps manage the itching in pruritus while detoxifying
- Hives
- Hypertension
- Immunization detox
- Injury

- Insect Bites
- Itching
- Keratoconjunctivitis sicca (Dry Eye)
- Metabolism Stimulator
- Osteoporosis
- Pituitary stimulations
- Sarcoptic mange
- Skin Inflammation
- Substitute for cortisone, antihistamines and other anti-inflammatory products
- Toxicity from drugs or medications
- Urethral obstruction (in male cats)
- Vaccination detox
- Wheezing
- Worms
- Wounds

Black Honeysuckle (Lonicera nigra)

- Kidney stones
- Mouth ulcers
- Stress

Black Poplar (Populus nigra)

- Tracheitis

Blackberry Vine (Rubus fructicosus)

- Ankylosing Spondylosis
- Chronic Interstitial Nephritis
- Intervertebral Disc Disease
- Joints
- Nephritis
- Obstructive Respiratory Disease
- Pain Relief
- Spondylitis

Bloodtwig Dogberry (Cornus sanguinea)

- Cancers of the thyroid gland
- Hematoma (post trauma)
- Hyperthyroid
- Hypothyroid

Briar Rose (Rosa canina)

- Abscess
- Canine Distemper
- Demodectic Mange
- Feline upper respiratory disease
- Immune Stimulator
- Infections
- Inflammation (chronic)

- Intervertebral Disc Disease
- Lyme's Disease
- Nasal congestion
- Nasal discharge
- Parvo (Canine)
- Pyometra
- Rhinitis
- Sneezing
- Spondylitis
- Tracheitis
- Upper Respiratory Illness
- Warts

Cedar of Lebanon (Cedrus libani)

- Allergies
- Dermatitis (chronic)
- Drainage, Skin/Kidney
- Mast Cell inhibitor

Christmas Holly (Ilex aquifolium)

- Epilepsy
- Renal Insufficiency
- Sclerosis, kidney

Common Birch (Betula pubescens)

- Bone Fractures

- Cataracts
- Hip Dysplasia
- Hepatitis
- Inflammation
- Injury
- Intervertebral Disc Disease
- Tooth (loose)
- Thrombosis
- Urea (elevated)
- Urethral obstruction (in male cats)
- Vaccination detox

Common Juniper (Juniperus communis)

- Aggressive behavior
- Attention Deficit Disorder
- Biliary Dysfunction
- Bladder infections
- Blood Pressure
- Cancer (Do not use in Kidney cancer)
- Cataracts
- Chemotherapy side effects
- Conjunctivitis
- Corneal disease
- Cystitis
- Demodectic Mange

- Diabetes
- Drainage, Kidney
- Drainage, Liver
- Feline Leukemia
- Fleas
- Fly Strike
- Heartworm
- Hepatitis
- Immunization detox
- Insect Bites
- Keratoconjunctivitis sicca (Dry Eye)
- Kidney drainer
- Kidney insufficiency
- Kidney stones
- Liver Drainer
- Mastitis
- Nephritis
- Polyarthritis
- Tendonitis
- Urethral obstruction (in male cats)
- Vaccination detox

Common Lilac (Syringa vulgaris)

- Heartworm

English Elm (Ulmus campestris)

- Corneal disease
- Ringworm
- Skin drainer
- Ulcerative Colitis
- Urea (elevated)
- Wounds

English Hawthorn (Crataegus oxyacantha)

- Arrhythmia
- Blood Pressure
- Cardiac insufficiency
- Cardiac spasms
- Cardiomyopathy
- Drainage, Arteries
- Edema, Pulmonary
- Edema, Cardiac
- Excellent regulator of slow cardiac movement
- Fibrillation
- Heart
- Heartworm
- Hypertension
- Increases myocardial tone (specific to the left side of the heart)
- Parvo (Canine)

- Pericardial pain
- Pulmonary Edema
- Tachycardia
- Thrombosis

European Alder (Alnus glutinosa)

- Allergic asthma
- Arterial emboli (stroke)
- Asthma
- Atrial Fibrillation
- Bleeding
- Bruising
- Burns
- Cystitis
- Drainage, Stomach
- Feline upper respiratory disease
- Fibrillation
- Heart
- Hives
- Inflammation (chronic)
- Memory
- Mouth ulcers
- Mucosa inflammation
- Osteomyelitis (bone infection)
- Peritonitis

- Rhinitis
- Sarcoptic mange
- Stroke
- Thrombosis
- Ulcers GI

European Ash (Fraxinus excelsior)

- Heartworm
- Kidney drainer
- Liver Drainer
- Synovial inflammation
- Wheezing
- Worms

European Beech (Fagus sylvatica)

- Kidney stones
- Obesity due to water retention
- Stimulates kidney function and urine output

European Chestnut (Castanea vesca)

- Drainage, Venous
- Edema, Lymphatic
- Lymphatic Drainer

European Filbert (Corylus avellana)

- Anemia
- Bruising
- Cough
- Drainage, Lung
- Kennel Cough
- Obstructive Respiratory Disease
- Pulmonary Fibrosis
- Upper Respiratory

European Grape Vine (Vitis vinifera)

- Ankylosing Spondylosis
- Arthritis
- Colitis
- Inflammation (chronic)

European Hornbeam (Carpinus betulus)

- Antitussive
- Choking cough
- Spasmodic and chronic rhinopharyngitis
- Tracheitis

European Oak (Quercus pedonculata)

- Addison's disease
- Anthelmintic (parasites)
- Enuresis
- Excellent for deficient adrenal glands
- Helps balance the adrenal gland and male hormones
- Strengthen the mucosa in periodontal disease
- Use on neutered males for hormonal balance secondary to castration

European Olive (Olea europaea)

- Arterial emboli (stroke)
- Blood Pressure
- Dementia
- Drainage, Arteries
- Heartworm
- Hypertension
- Kidney insufficiency
- Mastitis
- Obsessive/Compulsive Disease
- Phobias
- Renal Insufficiency
- Stroke
- Worms

European Walnut (Juglans regia)

- Abscess
- Acne
- Bloating
- Demodectic Mange
- Diabetes
- Diarrhea
- Diarrhea post-antibiotic
- Feline Distemper
- Flatulence
- Immune Stimulator
- Infections
- Insulin Balancer
- Intestinal parasites
- Lyme's Disease

Fig Tree (Ficus carica)

- Acute or chronic diarrhea
- Acute or chronic vomiting
- All gastrointestinal illness
- Bloating
- Colitis
- Concussion

- Constipation
- Cough
- Diabetes
- Diarrhea
- Drainage, Liver
- Drainage, Nervous system
- Drainage, Stomach
- Eosinophilic Granuloma
- Feline Distemper
- Flatulence
- Hematoma (post-trauma)
- Intestinal parasites
- Irritable Bowel Syndrome
- Kennel Cough
- Mucosa digestive
- Parvo (Canine)
- Stress
- Thymus regulator
- Ulcerative Colitis
- Ulcers GI
- Vomiting
- Warts

Giant Redwood (Sequoia gigantea)

- Aging

- Bone Fractures
- Breeding
- Enuresis
- Immune Stimulator
- Improves endurance
- Joints
- Lyme's Disease
- Osteoporosis
- Pain relief
- Paresis and paralysis of the rear limbs
- Prostatitis
- Urinary incontinence
- Urinary system
- Weakness of anything below the waist of an animal

Hedge Maple (Acer campestre)

- Antifungal
- Antiviral
- Diabetes
- Thrombosis

Lemon Bark (Citrus limonum)

- Insomnia
- Liver Drainer

Lime Tree (Tilia tomentosa)

- Aggressive behavior
- Analgesic (pain)
- Anxiety
- Arterial emboli (stroke)
- Attention Deficit Disorder
- Canine Distemper
- Colitis
- Depression
- Drainage, Nervous system
- Epilepsy
- Fear
- Hyperactivity
- Hypertension
- Insomnia
- Irritability
- Mucosa inflammation
- Neurological diseases
- Phobias
- Rabies Miasm
- Vaccine-related neurological disease
- Very effective in calming the nervous system

Lithy Tree (Viburnum lantana)

- Allergic asthma
- Asthma
- Canine Distemper
- Cough
- Deafness
- Drainage, Lung
- Feline Leukemia
- Hyperthyroidism
- Kennel Cough
- Lung Drainer
- Thyroid hyperactive
- Tinnitus
- Tracheitis
- Upper Respiratory
- Vertigo

Maize (Zea mais)

- Heart
- Kidney Drainer
- Lung Drainer

Mistletoe (Viscum album)

- Mastitis

- Panic attacks
- Tinnitus
- Tumors, growth inhibitors
- Urea (elevated)

Mountain Pine (Pinus montana)

- Arthritis
- Cartilage regeneration
- Degenerative arthritis
- Degenerative myelopathy
- Disc-related paralysis
- Excellent remedy for spinal problems
- Hives
- Intervetebral Disc Disease
- Joints
- Osteoporosis
- Pain Relief
- Spinal trauma
- Spondylitis
- Spondylosis
- Tendon Repair

Prim Wort (Ligustrum vulgare)

- Ringworm
- Skin Drainer

- Tinnitus
- Vertigo

Raspberry (Rubus idaeus)

- Attention Deficit Disorder
- Delivery (birth)
- Dysmenorrhoea
- Hyperfolliculinism
- Inhibiting effect on the anterior lobe of the pituitary
- Parturition (whelping)
- Pyometra
- Regulates ovarian secretion
- Retained Placenta
- Wounds

Red Alder (Alnus incana)

- Anaphylaxis
- Heart
- Thrombosis
- Tracheitis

Red Spruce (Abies pectinata)

- Osteomyelitis (bone infection)

Rosemary (Rosmarinus officinalis)

- Action specifically for the gallbladder
- Biliary colic
- Biliary dyskinesia with hyper- or hypotonia
- Breeding
- Chronic cholecystitis
- Colitis
- Dementia
- Depression
- Drainage, Gallbladder
- Drainage, Liver
- Excellent anti-spasmodic
- Hypertension
- Memory
- Minor hepatic insufficiency
- Obsessive/Compulsive Disorder
- Prostatitis
- Regulates gall bladder motility
- Vertigo

Rowan Tree (Sorbus domestica)

- Assists the body in clearing out toxins
- Chronic choking conditions
- Chronic Otitis

- Drainage, Venous
- Deafness
- Ears, Nose, Throat conditions
- Feline Leukemia
- Hearing loss
- Mastitis
- Nasal discharge
- Pain Relief
- Tinnitus
- Tonsillitis
- Vertigo

Rye Grain (Secale cereale)

- Acne
- Chronic skin conditions
- Dermis repair
- Hepatitis
- Liver Drainer
- Ringworm
- Skin repair

Silver Birch (Betula verrucosa)

- Bladder infections
- Bladder Stones
- Blood Urea Nitrogen

- Caries/Dental decay
- Ear, Nose and Throat
- Hepatitis
- Kidney drainer
- Nephritis
- Osteomyelitis (bone infection)
- Urea (elevated)

Sweet Almond (Prunus amygdalus)

- Anemia
- Amylidosis (Kidney)
- Hypothyroidism
- Obsessive Compulsive Disease
- Phobias
- Renal Amylidosis
- Thrombosis
- Thyroid hypoactive
- Urea (elevated)

Tamarisk (Tamarix gallica)

- Anemia
- Thrombin formation regulator
- Thrombocytopenia

Wild Woodvine (Ampelopsis weitchii)

- Anterior cruciate ruptures
- Degenerative arthritis, cartilage damage
- Hip dysplasia
- Joint-related problems
- Sprains/strains
- Tendon Repair
- Trauma

Wine Berry (Vaccinum vitis idaea)

- Aging
- Balancing hormones
- Bladder infections
- Colitis
- Constipation
- Diarrhea
- Drainage, Bladder
- Drainage, Intestines
- Irritable Bowel Syndrome
- Joints
- Kidney oxalo-calcic stones
- Mucosa digestive
- Nephritis
- Pain relief
- Parvo (Canine)

- Prostatitis
- Pulmonary Fibrosis
- Pyometra
- Spayed dogs and cats
- Thyroid adenoma
- Ulcerative Colitis
- Urea (elevated)
- Urinary infection
- Vaginal discharge (leukorrhea)
- Weight after surgery (in spayed animals)
- Youth revitalized (in spayed animals)

Gemmotherapy Remedies
(Botanical Name)

Abies pectinata (Red Spruce)

- Osteomyelitis (bone infection)

Acer campestre (Hedge Maple)

- Antifungal
- Antiviral
- Diabetes
- Thrombosis

Alnus glutinosa (European Alder)

- Allergic asthma
- Arterial emboli (stroke)
- Asthma
- Atrial Fibrillation
- Bleeding
- Bruising
- Burns
- Cystitis
- Drainage, Stomach

- Feline upper-respiratory disease
- Fibrillation
- Heart
- Hives
- Inflammation (chronic)
- Memory
- Mouth ulcers
- Mucosa inflammation
- Osteomyelitis (bone infection)
- Peritonitis
- Rhinitis
- Sarcoptic mange
- Stroke
- Thrombosis
- Ulcers, Gastro-Intestinal Tract

Alnus incana (Red Alder)

- Anaphylaxis
- Heart
- Thrombosis
- Tracheitis

Ampelopsis weitchii (Wild Woodvine)

- Anterior cruciate ruptures

- Degenerative arthritis, cartilage damage
- Hip dysplasia
- Joint-related problems
- Sprains/strains
- Tendon Repair
- Trauma

Betula pubescens (Common Birch)

- Bone Fractures
- Cataracts
- Hip Dysplasia
- Hepatitis
- Inflammation
- Injury
- Intervertebral Disc Disease
- Tooth (loose)
- Thrombosis
- Urea (elevated)
- Urethral obstruction (in male cats)
- Vaccination detox

Betula verrucosa (Silver Birch)

- Bladder infections
- Bladder Stones
- Blood Urea Nitrogen

- Caries/Dental decay
- Ear, Nose and Throat
- Hepatitis
- Kidney drainer
- Nephritis
- Osteomyelitis (bone infection)
- Urea (elevated)

Carpinus betulus (European Hornbeam)

- Spasmodic and chronic rhinopharyngitis
- Tracheitis
- Antitussive
- Choking cough

Castanea vesca (European Chestnut)

- Drainage, Venous
- Edema, Lymphatic
- Lymphatic Drainer

Cedrus libani (Cedar of Lebanon)

- Allergies
- Dermatitis (chronic)
- Drainage, Skin/Kidney
- Mast Cell inhibitor

Citrus limonum (Lemon Bark)

- Insomnia
- Liver Drainer

Cornus sanguinea (Bloodtwig Dogberry)

- Hematoma (post-trauma)
- Hyperthyroid
- Hypothyroid
- Cancers of the thyroid gland

Corylus avellana (European Filbert)

- Anemia
- Bruising
- Cough
- Drainage, Lung
- Kennel Cough
- Obstructive Respiratory Disease
- Pulmonary Fibrosis
- Upper Respiratory

Crataegus oxyacantha (English Hawthorn)

- Excellent regulator of slow cardiac movement

- Increases myocardial tone (specific to the left side of the heart)
- Arrhythmia
- Blood Pressure
- Cardiac insufficiency
- Cardiomyopathy
- Cardiac spasms
- Drainage, Arteries
- Edema, Cardiac
- Edema, Pulmonary
- Fibrillation
- Heart
- Heartworm
- Hypertension
- Parvo (Canine)
- Pericardial pain
- Pulmonary Edema
- Tachycardia
- Thrombosis

Fagus sylvatica (European Beech)

- Stimulates kidney function and urine output
- Kidney stones
- Obesity due to water retention

Ficus carica (Fig Tree)

- All gastrointestinal illness
- Acute or chronic diarrhea
- Acute or chronic vomiting
- Bloating
- Colitis
- Concussion
- Constipation
- Cough
- Diabetes
- Diarrhea
- Drainage, Liver
- Drainage, Nervous system
- Drainage, Stomach
- Eosinophilic Granuloma
- Feline Distemper
- Flatulence
- Hematoma (post-trauma)
- Irritable Bowel Syndrome
- Intestinal parasites
- Kennel Cough
- Mucosa digestive
- Parvo (Canine)
- Stress
- Thymus regulator

- Ulcers GI
- Ulcerative Colitis
- Vomiting
- Warts

Fraxinus excelsior (European Ash)

- Heartworm
- Kidney drainer
- Liver Drainer
- Synovial inflammation
- Wheezing
- Worms

Ilex aquifolium (Christmas Holly)

- Epilepsy
- Renal Insufficiency
- Sclerosis, kidney

Juglans regia (European Walnut)

- Abscess
- Acne
- Bloating
- Demodectic Mange
- Diabetes

- Diarrhea
- Diarrhea post-antibiotic
- Feline Distemper
- Flatulence
- Immune Stimulator
- Infections
- Insulin Balancer
- Intestinal parasites
- Lyme's Disease

Juniperus communis (Common Juniper)

- Aggressive behavior
- Attention Deficit Disorder
- Biliary Dysfunction
- Bladder infections
- Blood Pressure
- Cancer (Do not use in Kidney cancer)
- Cataracts
- Chemotherapy side effects
- Conjunctivitis
- Corneal disease
- Cystitis
- Demodectic Mange
- Diabetes
- Drainage, Kidney

- Drainage, Liver
- Feline Leukemia
- Fleas
- Fly Strike
- Heartworm
- Hepatitis
- Immunization detox
- Insect Bites
- Keratoconjunctivitis sicca (Dry Eye)
- Kidney drainer
- Kidney insufficiency
- Kidney stones
- Liver Drainer
- Mastitis
- Nephritis
- Polyarthritis
- Tendonitis
- Urethral obstruction (in male cats)
- Vaccination detox

Ligustrum vulgare (Prim Wort)

- Ringworm
- Skin Drainer
- Tinnitus
- Vertigo

Lonicera nigra (Black Honeysuckle)

- Kidney stones
- Mouth ulcers
- Stress

Olea europaea (European Olive)

- Arterial emboli (stroke)
- Blood Pressure
- Dementia
- Drainage, Arteries
- Heartworm
- Hypertension
- Kidney insufficiency
- Mastitis
- Obsessive/Compulsive Disease
- Phobias
- Renal Insufficiency
- Stroke
- Worms

Pinus montana (Mountain Pine)

- Degenerative arthritis
- Degenerative myelopathy

- Disc-related paralysis
- Excellent remedy for spinal problems
- Spinal trauma
- Spondylosis
- Arthritis
- Cartilage regeneration
- Hives
- Intervertebral Disc Disease
- Joints
- Osteoporosis
- Pain Relief
- Spondylitis
- Tendon Repair

Populus nigra (Black Poplar)

- Tracheitis

Prunus amygdalus (Sweet Almond)

- Anemia
- Amylidosis (Kidney)
- Hypothyroidism
- Obsessive Compulsive Disease
- Phobias
- Renal Amylidosis
- Thrombosis

- Thyroid hypoactive
- Urea (elevated)

Quercus pedonculata (European Oak)

- Addison's disease
- Anthelmintic (parasites)
- Enuresis
- Excellent for deficient adrenal glands
- Helps balance the adrenal gland and male hormones.
- Strengthen the mucosa in periodontal disease
- Use on neutered males for hormonal balance secondary to castration

Ribes nigrum (Black Currant)

- Adrenal failure
- Adrenal imbalance-strengthens the adrenal glands
- Allergic conditions
- Substitute for cortisone, antihistamines and other anti-inflammatory products
- Helps manage the itching in pruritus while detoxifying
- Balances the animal's immune system
- Asthma
- Anaphylaxis

- Bites and Stings
- Blood Urea Nitrogen
- Conjunctivitis
- Corneal disease
- Corticosteroid alternative
- Ear, Nose and Throat
- Fleas
- Heartworm
- Hives
- Hypertension
- Immunization detox
- Injury
- Insect Bites
- Itching
- Keratoconjunctivitis sicca (Dry Eye)
- Metabolism Stimulator
- Osteoporosis
- Pituitary stimulations
- Sarcoptic mange
- Skin Inflammation
- Toxicity from drugs or medications
- Urethral obstruction (in male cats)
- Vaccination detox
- Wheezing
- Worms
- Wounds

Rosa canina (Briar Rose)

- Abscess
- Canine Distemper
- Demodectic Mange
- Feline upper-respiratory disease
- Immune Stimulator
- Infections
- Inflammation (chronic)
- Intervertebral Disc Disease
- Lyme's Disease
- Nasal congestion
- Nasal discharge
- Parvo (Canine)
- Pyometra
- Rhinitis
- Spondylitis
- Sneezing
- Tracheitis
- Upper-Respiratory Illness
- Warts

Rosmarinus officinalis (Rosemary)

- Action specifically for the gallbladder
- Excellent anti-spasmodic

- Regulates gall bladder motility
- Minor hepatic insufficiency
- Biliary dyskinesia with hyper- or hypotonia
- Biliary colic
- Chronic cholecystitis
- Breeding
- Colitis
- Dementia
- Depression
- Drainage, Gallbladder
- Drainage, Liver
- Hypertension
- Memory
- Obsessive/Compulsive Disorder
- Prostatitis
- Vertigo

Rubus fructicosus (Blackberry Vine)

- Ankylosing Spondylitis
- Chronic Interstitial Nephritis
- Intervertebral Disc Disease
- Joints
- Nephritis
- Obstructive Respiratory Disease
- Pain Relief

- Spondylitis

Rubus idaeus (Raspberry)

- Attention Deficit Disorder
- Delivery
- Dysmenorrhoea
- Hyperfolliculinism
- Inhibiting effect on the anterior lobe of the pituitary
- Parturition (whelping)
- Pyometra
- Retained Placenta
- Wounds

Secale cereale (Rye Grain)

- Acne
- Chronic skin conditions
- Dermis repair
- Hepatitis
- Liver Drainer
- Ringworm
- Skin repair

Sequoia gigantea (Giant Redwood)

- Aging

- Bone Fractures
- Breeding
- Enuresis
- Immune Stimulator
- Improves endurance
- Joints
- Lyme's Disease
- Osteoporosis
- Pain relief
- Prostatitis
- Paresis and paralysis of the rear limbs
- Urinary incontinence
- Urinary system
- Weakness of anything below the waist of an animal

Sorbus domestica (Rowan Tree)

- Assists the body in clearing out toxins
- Chronic choking conditions
- Chronic Otitis
- Drainage, Venous
- Deafness
- Ears, Nose, Throat conditions
- Feline Leukemia
- Hearing loss
- Mastitis

- Nasal discharge
- Pain Relief
- Tinnitus
- Tonsillitis
- Vertigo

Syringa vulgaris (Common Lilac)

- Heartworm

Tamarix gallica (Tamarisk)

- Anemia
- Thrombin formation regulator
- Thrombocytopenia

Tilia tomentosa (Lime Tree)

- Aggressive behavior
- Analgesic (pain)
- Anxiety
- Arterial emboli (stroke)
- Attention Deficit Disorder
- Canine Distemper
- Colitis
- Depression
- Drainage, Nervous System

- Epilepsy
- Fear
- Hyperactivity

- Hypertension
- Insomnia
- Irritability
- Mucosa inflammation
- Neurological diseases
- Phobias
- Rabies Miasm
- Very effective in calming the nervous system
- Vaccine-related neurological disease

Ulmus campestris (English Elm)

- Corneal disease
- Ringworm
- Skin drainer
- Ulcerative Colitis
- Urea (elevated)
- Wounds

Vaccinum vitis idaea (Wine Berry)

- Aging
- Bladder infections

- Colitis
- Constipation
- Diarrhea
- Drainage, Bladder
- Drainage, Intestines
- Irritable Bowel Syndrome
- Joints
- Kidney oxalo-calcic stones
- Mucosa digestive
- Nephritis
- Pain relief
- Parvo (Canine)
- Prostatitis
- Pulmonary Fibrosis
- Pyometra
- Spayed dogs and cats
- Thyroid adenoma
- Ulcerative Colitis
- Urea (elevated)
- Urinary infection
- Vaginal discharge (leukorrhea)
- Balancing hormones
- Weight after surgery (in spayed animals)
- Youth revitalizer (in spayed animals)

Viburnum lantana (Lithy Tree)

- Allergic asthma
- Asthma
- Canine Distemper
- Cough
- Deafness
- Drainage, Lung
- Feline Leukemia
- Hyperthyroidism
- Kennel Cough
- Lung Drainer
- Thyroid hyperactive
- Tinnitus
- Tracheitis
- Upper Respiratory
- Vertigo

Viscum album (Mistletoe)

- Mastitis
- Tinnitus
- Panic attacks
- Tumors, growth inhibitors
- Urea (elevated)

Vitis vinifera (European Grape Vine)

- Ankylosing Spondylosis
- Arthritis
- Colitis
- Inflammation (chronic)

Zea mais (Maize)

- Heart
- Kidney Drainer
- Lung Drainer

Gemmotherapy Materia Medica

Black Currant (Ribes nigrum)
All allergic conditions will benefit from the use of this Gemmotherapy remedy. Good for itching or scratching. It helps support the adrenal glands and has anti-inflammatory properties. This remedy can also be used topically on areas of inflammation of the skin.

Black Poplar (Populus nigra)
The action of this Gemmotherapy remedy is helpful when the animal's nutritional reserves are depleted by diarrhea or watery stools. Black Poplar is a short term remedy and should only be used four to five weeks maximum to protect the liver.

Bloodtwig Dogberry (Cornus sanguinea)
Hypo- or Hyper-thyroidism is helped by this particular Gemmotherapy remedy. Helps to detoxify and strengthen the thyroid gland.

Briar Rose (aka Dog Rose) (Rosa canina)
Used for any nasal conditions such as sneezing, congestion or discharge. It detoxifies the mucus membranes of the nasal passages and sinuses.

Common Birch (Betula pubescens)
Common Birch helps eliminate uric acid. Used in the treatment of rheumatism, kidney disorders, and skin problems. Common Birch helps to stimulate the endocrine system, and is an excellent liver and kidney drainer. Has an anti-inflammatory effect on the body. Used in the treatment of osteoarthritis. Good for detoxification of the body after vaccination. It is referred to as the universal drainer for the entire body. I often use it alone in cases where the animal is in need of a gentle multi-system drainer. It is a strong stimulant for the immune system and effective against colds, flu, pharyngitis and all upper-respiratory diseases. It is my favorite remedy for hip-joint issues; such as hip dysplasia, arthritis, and degenerative conditions of the hip joints. It stimulates local vascularization to the hip area and stimulates osteoblastic action to help slow down or repair arthritic conditions.

Common Juniper (Juniperus communis)
This Gemmotherapy remedy is useful for the very deficient liver in the phase of decompensation, jaundice, and various types of cirrhosis. Main drainer for the kidney and liver, especially where there is an auto-immune component. Anti-inflammatory for the liver and secondarily as a diuretic for the kidney. It is recommended not to use more than six weeks daily due to potential fatigue-causing if used for too long a period

of time. I recommend once per day in the small doses indicated in the book and then weekly thereafter for maintenance. **It can be used to treat all tumors and cancers except for cancer of the kidney.**

English Elm (Ulmus campestris)
Useful for skin ailments, such as skin infections and acne. It is an excellent drainer for the kidney and liver. Also, a good remedy for gout and skin infections such as: eczema, acne, herpes, psoriasis and ulcerations of the extremities.

English Hawthorn (Crataegus oxyacantha)
Regulator of cardiac movement, when it is slow. Increases myocardial tone, in particular to the left side of the heart. Has a sedative effect on all pericardial pain. Indicated in cardiac insufficiency and associated symptoms, cardiac spasms, tachycardia and arrhythmias as well as in pericardial pain. Excellent for regulating blood pressure, anti-thrombotic effect. Reduces congestive heart failure and pulmonary edema symptoms. Helps to stabilize the electro-conductive activity of the heart. It works well in conjunction with Cornus sanguinea (Bloodtwig) which helps to protect the heart from myocardial infarction. It is excellent remedy for the arteries of the heart.

European Alder (Alnus glutinosa)
The action of this Gemmotherapy remedy is helpful for allergic asthma. This is an excellent remedy for inflammatory conditions originating in the mucosa. It is an excellent remedy to use for stroke cases due its collateral circulation activity. Cerebral and coronary obstructions will heal more efficiently with the use of this remedy by helping the body create by-pass vascularization to re-establish a new collateral circulation.

European Beech (Fagus sylvatica)
Stimulates renal function and urine output. Indicated in renal lithiasis, renal insufficiency and in obesity due to water retention. It is indicated for any sclerotic condition of the lung. It can be used to reduce cholesterol, uric acid and urea.

European Grape Vine (Vitis vinifera)
Indicated in very painful, deforming rheumatism and in arthritis affecting the small joints. Useful for any chronic inflammatory condition of the joints. Recommended in colitis, to help with the detoxification and healing process.

European Hornbeam (Carpinus betulus)
Active in the rhinopharynx and trachea, ensuring healing of damaged mucosal surfaces and relieving spasm.

Indicated for spasmodic and chronic rhinopharyngitis, tracheitis and tracheo-bronchitis. Is antitussive. Drainer for the pharynx and surrounding tissues. It is often referred to as the ear, nose and throat remedy. It is very specific for the mucosa of the entire respiratory system. Remedy for treating emphysema in people. Also it is used in thrombocytopenia by normalizing the blood's ability to clot.

European Oak (Quercus pedonculata)
Oak is excellent for restoring vitality in male animals. Excellent to use in neutered male animals that have a sluggish metabolism secondary to loss of male hormone production by stimulating the cortex of the adrenal gland.

European Olive (Olea europaea)
Provides the appropriate balance of phospholipids necessary for proper brain functioning. Is also known for heart strengthening. Excellent for cleaning out the blood vessels through out the body. Helps prevent and treats any vascular obstructive situation, especially strokes. Used to lower cholesterol and balance lipids in the blood. Helps break down scar tissue in the arterial supply to the brain and is indicated for treating Alzheimer's disease or other memory-loss conditions. Good in phobic conditions, compulsive disorders and anxiety. **IT IS NOT RECOMMENDED**

FOR CANCER PATIENTS DUE TO THE ANTISCLEROTIC PROPERTIES OF THE REMEDY, WHICH MEANS IT WOULD BREAK DOWN THE SCAR TISSUE LIMITING THE SPREAD OF THE CANCER.

European Walnut (Juglans regia)
Useful in diabetes to help balance the blood sugars. Exceptional for pancreas function and helps regenerate this organ during and after pancreatitis attacks. It is excellent for chronic inflammatory conditions of the skin, liver and any mucus membrane. Excellent long-term treatment for chronic streptococcus or staphylococcus infections and infections of the mucosa in the trachea and bronchial aspects of the lungs. Good for antibiotic-induced diarrhea, for restoring the intestinal flora and for malabsorption conditions of the gut, secondary to pancreatic insufficiencies. It helps to normalize pancreatic production of enzymes and insulin. It is excellent for cleaning the insulin receptor sites and helping balance the blood sugar of an animal with diabetes. It is also very good for infections of the gallbladder.

Fig Tree (Ficus carica)
All gastrointestinal-related disease will be helped by the use of Fig Tree. Administer this remedy at feeding time or in food to detoxify and strengthen the intestinal tract.

Excellent for any gastrointestinal issues your animal may be dealing with and for protecting the GI system from toxic materials they may ingest. It is excellent for ulceration of stomach and duodenum. Good for inflammation of the esophagus. Helps balance digestive enzymes and acid production of the GI system as well as having a healing effect on the mucus membranes. Indicated for intracranial hematomas secondary to trauma. Indicated for eosinophilic granuloma and to help regulate the thymus gland.

Giant Redwood (Sequoia gigantea)
For weakness of limbs, urinary or fecal incontinence, prostatitis and/or lethargy. It is the precursor of estrogen and excellent for spayed females with hormone deficiency secondary to the removal of their ovaries and uterus. **IT IS NOT INDICATED FOR PROSTATE CANCER.** It is indicated for acute prostatitis, fibroids, dysmenorrhea and osteoporosis. Indicated for semi-spontaneous fractures (glass-bone disease). Gives the patient a sense of well being.

Hedge Maple (Acer campestre)
Improves digestion, and has a detoxifying effect on kidneys. Lowers rate of blood sugar, and is therefore useful in the treatment of diabetes. Excellent for any viral infections, fatigue and fibromyalgia. It is also indicated for the treatment of gallstones and prevention.

Good for anticipatory fears which are ill-defined.

Lime Tree (Tilia tomentosa)
This is very effective in calming the nervous system so the animal can act instead of react. Lime Tree will complement any form of seizure therapy. Excellent for detoxing and helping repair any part of the nervous system. Excellent for insomnia and for relaxing nervous patients. I recommend starting with a low dose and working up to effect. If the patient feels too sleepy, reduce the dose by half, and half again, until you find the desired optimal effect. Useful for headaches, migraines and neuralgia. Good for anticipatory fears that are ill-defined by the patient. I use it in all my epilepsy cases.

Lithy Tree (Viburnum lantana)
Use for treating chronic allergies. Useful as a powerful lung-draining remedy and helps to restore the lung to its optimal health. Indicated for treating chronic rhinitis, allergies, eczema and asthma from different causes. Good choice for spasmodic conditions of the bronchi. I use this remedy in all my lung cases, no matter what the cause may be, with excellent results.

Mountain Pine (Pinus montana)
Will strengthen and detoxify the spine and any small joint-related problems. Excellent for any form of arthritis,

regardless of location. It has a regenerative action on bones, cartilage, ligaments and tendons. It also is helpful in the healing process of arteries and lymphatic system. It can be used in osteoporosis along with Rosa canina (Briar Rose).

Prim Wort (Ligustrum vulgare)
Helps facilitate drainage of the skin, mucus membrane and the kidneys. Is useful in chronic intestinal conditions. Can be used for colitis, infections of the mouth, ulcerations of the legs and bedsores. Other uses are tonsillitis, bronchitis, intestinal and uterine bleeding and vaginal discharges.

Raspberry (Rubus idaeus)
It is very good for conditions involving the pelvic region of females. I use it for whelping for the discomfort of birthing and estrus. Excellent for any uterine or vaginal discharges. Indicated for endometrial hyperplasia and post whelping to help clean out the uterus. Excellent for retained placenta or to help the female with the release of the placenta after birthing occurs. Helps females who are slow to develop reproductively. Has an inhibiting effect on the anterior lobe of the pituitary and in particular regulates ovarian secretion. Indicated in syndromes with hyperfolliculinism and in dysmenorrhea.

Rosemary (Rosmarinus officinalis)
The action of this Gemmotherapy remedy is specifically oriented towards the liver and gallbladder. An excellent anti-spasmodic which regulates gallbladder motility. Indicated in minor hepatic insufficiency, biliary dyskinesia with hyper- or hypotonia, biliary colic and chronic cholecystitis. *I have found it to be the premier remedy for any form of jaundice.* Can help in minimizing the animal's biological aging process. Excellent choice in animals that seem to be getting old prematurely. Indicated for prostatitis and reproductive insufficiencies both in females and males. Good choice for colitis due to its effect on the intestinal mucosa and is suggested for colitis. Can be used for chronic nervousness. IT CAN BE USED LONG TERM BUT DUE TO ITS EUPHORIC ACTION, **HIGH DOSES COULD PRODUCE EPILEPTIC CONDITIONS IF THE PATIENT IS SO PREDISPOSED.** I DO NOT USE THIS REMEDY ON ANY PATIENT WHO HAS ANY SEIZURING HISTORY. I HAVE NEVER HAD A NON-SEIZURING PATIENT HAVE ANY ILL EFFECTS FROM TAKING THIS REMEDY AS PER MY INSTRUCTIONS PRESENTED IN THIS BOOK.

Rowan Tree (Sorbus domestica)
Useful for ear, nose and throat conditions. My
first choice for ear infections of any kind, especially
those following vaccination. Main remedy used for
cleaning out the veins of the body. Good for congestion
of the veins, restless-leg syndrome, tinnitus, deafness,
strong drainer for the lymphatic system, and brain
tumors. If your animal has any chronic ear
infection, NEVER VACCINATE IT, EVER. These
animals are very sensitive to the side effects of vaccines
and will surely deteriorate if you continue to vaccinate
them. Note: On the vaccine insert, it states: "Only
vaccinate healthy animals." Therefore, any animal with
a chronic medical condition is NOT HEALTHY.

Rye Grain (Secale cereale)
Used for any chronic skin conditions to help detoxify the
skin and liver of animals with chronic dermatitis
conditions. It is also indicated for acute and chronic
forms of hepatitis with jaundice. Useful for psoriasis.

Silver Birch (Betula pendula)
An excellent liver and kidney drainer. Indicated as an
anti-inflammatory, useful in the treatment of
osteoarthritis. It is known for its regenerative potential,
especially in bones. It is recommended to alternate with
Red Spruce (Abies pectinata) in the treatment of
juvenile osteochondritis, chronic osteomyelitis, and

infant dental caries. I use it the treatment of kidney failure, albuminuria, nephritis, hepatitis, pancreatitis and splenic disorders.

Tamarisk (Tamarix gallica)
Active on the red-cell series, stimulating erythrocyte formation. Indicated in hypochromic anemia. I use it in all thrombocytopenia and bleeding disorders. I also use it in cases of non-regenerative anemia, especially those secondary to kidney failure. You can also use it in conjunction with Fig Tree (Ficus carica), to treat eosinophilic granulomas. Also a powerful stimulant for the bone marrow. SHOULD NOT BE USED WITH PATIENTS WITH ARTERIOSCLEROSIS.

Wild Woodvine (Ampelopsis weitchii)
Useful for any joint-related problems such as: hip dysplasia, anterior cruciate ruptures, sprains/strains, degenerative arthritis, and cartilage damage. I use it in ankylosing spondylitis and for any joint injury, no matter what the cause may be. This remedy is recommended for detoxification and helping regenerate ligaments, cartilage and bone. It works very well in conjunction with Mountain Pine (Pinus montana) to help in the healing and discomfort of joint injuries.

Wine Berry (Vaccinum vitis idaea)
Wine Berry is excellent for helping to balance
hormones. Especially first-rate in spayed animals where
they have gained weight after surgery. I have found this
particular Gemmotherapy remedy can bring back the
youth of the animal before it was spayed. It is excellent
for necrosis of the toes and fingers in diabetes, diabetic
gangrene and has its major effect on the small arteries
and arterioles. It can help with hyalinated ovaries,
benign hyaline tumors: uterine fibromas and adenomas
of the thyroid, renal glomerular hyalinization and
pulmonary emboli. Excellent remedy for aging and for
maximizing the animal's biological clock. It is another
remedy that is indicated for colitis, diarrhea and
colibacillosis. It is also indicated for osteoporosis due to
its effect on calcium metabolism and absorption. It is
also excellent for colon-related problems, such as lack
of colon motility. It acts as a stimulant to the colon to
help with the lack of bowel motility. In hyperactive,
spasmodic-colon situations it acts as a sedative and
antispasmodic. It also reduces uric acid, urea and
cholesterol. Useful as a disinfectant for the urinary and
intestinal system. Excellent for recurring urinary
infections in females. It also has a place in
treating nephritis, viral pericarditis and rheumatoid
arthritis.

Common Conditions and the Gemmotherapy Remedies

Used to Treat Them

Abscess......................European Walnut (any infection)

Abscess (newborn).....Briar Rose

Acne..........................European Walnut (any infection)

.................................Rye Grain (chronic acne)

Adrenal failure or imbalance

.................................Black Currant (adrenal gland)

.................................European Oak (adrenal cortex)

Aging........................Wine Berry, Giant Redwood and

.................................Rosemary

Aggressive behavior...Lime Tree, Common Juniper

Allergic asthma...........Black Currant, Lithy Tree,

.................................European Alder

Allergies....................Black Currant, Rosemary

.................................Cedar of Lebanon,

Amylidosis (Kidney) ... Sweet Almond, Common Juniper

Anemia...................... Tamarisk, European Filbert

Analgesic (pain).. .... Lime Tree

Anaphylaxis .... Black Currant, Red Alder

Ankylosing Spondylosis

.... European Grape Vine,

.... Mountain Pine, Blackberry Vine

Antifungal................... Hedge Maple

Anthelmintic (parasites)

.... European Oak

Antiviral...................... Hedge Maple

Anxiety....................... Lime Tree

Arrhythmia .... English Hawthorn

Arterial emboli (stroke)

.... Lime Tree, European Alder,

.... European Olive

Arthritis ....European Grape Vine, Common

...............................Juniper, Wild Woodvine and

...............................Mountain Pine

Asthma ....Black Currant, Lithy Tree,

...............................European Alder

Atrial Fibrillation..........European Alder

Attention Deficit Disorder

...............................Lime Tree, Common Juniper

Biliary Dysfunction......Rosemary, Common Juniper

Bites and Stings ....Black Currant

Bladder infections.......Silver Birch, Wine Berry,

...............................Common Juniper

Bladder Stones...........Silver Birch

Bleeding ....European Alder

Bloating ....European Walnut, Fig Tree

Blood Pressure...........English Hawthorn, European

...............................Olive, Common Juniper

Blood Urea Nitrogen...Black Currant, Common Juniper,

...............................Silver Birch

Bone Fractures .... Common Birch, Giant Redwood

Breeding .... Oak, Giant Redwood,

.... Black Currant

Bruising .... European Alder, European Filbert

Burns .... European Alder

Canine Distemper ...... Fig Free, Lithy Tree, Lime Tree,

.... Briar Rose

Caries/Dental decay... Silver Birch

Cancer   .... Common Juniper (DO NOT use

.... in Kidney cancer)

Cardiomyopathy .... European Hawthorn

Cartilage regeneration

.... Wild Woodvine, Mountain Pine

Cataracts .... Common Juniper, Common Birch

Chemotherapy side effects

.... Common Juniper

Chronic Interstitial Nephritis

.... European Beech, BlackberryVine

Choking cough .... European Hornbeam

Colitis..........................Fig Tree, Rosemary, Lime Tree,

...............................European Grape Vine, WineBerry

Concussion.................Fig Tree

Conjunctivitis ....Common Juniper, Black Currant

Constipation ....Fig Tree, Wine Berry

Corneal disease ....Common Juniper, Black Currant

...............................Black Popular, Raspberry,

...............................English Elm

Corticosteroid alternative

...............................Black Currant

Cough   ....Fig Tree, Walnut, Lithy Tree,

...............................European Filbert

Cystitis   ....Common Juniper,

...............................European Alder

Deafness ....Rowan Tree, Lithy Tree

Delivery ....Raspberry

Dementia...................Rosemary and European Olive

Demodectic Mange ....Common Juniper, Briar Rose,

...............................European Walnut

Depression................. Lime Tree, Rosemary **(not to be**

.... **used in epileptics)**

Dermatitis Chronic ..... Cedar of Lebanon

Dermis repair .... Rye Grain

Diabetes.................... European Walnut, Fig Tree,

.... Hedge Maple, Common Juniper

Diarrhea.................... Fig Tree, Wine Berry,

.... European Walnut

Diarrhea post-antibiotic

.... European Walnut

Drainage, Arteries...... European Hawthorn,

.... European Olive

Drainage, Bladder...... Wine Berry

Drainage, Gallbladder Rosemary

Drainage, Heart .... European Hawthorn

Drainage, Intestines... Wine Berry

Drainage, Kidney .... Common Juniper,

.... Common Birch,

.... Cedar of Lebanon

Drainage, Liver ....Common Juniper, Rosemary,

...................................Fig Tree

Drainage, Lung...........Lithy Tree, European Filbert

Drainage, Nervous system

...................................Lime Tree, Fig Tree

Drainage, Skin............Cedar of Lebanon, English Elm

Drainage, Stomach.....Fig Tree, European Alder

Drainage, Venous.......Rowan Tree, European Chestnut

Ear, Nose and Throat .Rowan Tree, Briar Rose,

...................................European Hornbeam

...................................Black Currant, Silver Birch

Edema, Cardiac..........European Hawthorn

Edema, Lymphatic......European Chestnut

Edema, Pulmonary.....European Hawthorn

Enuresis ....Giant Redwood, European Oak

Eosinophilic Granuloma

...................................Fig Tree

Epilepsy......................Lime Tree, Holly Tree

Fear............................Lime Tree

Feline upper-respiratory disease

.... Briar Rose, European Alder

Feline Distemper........ Fig Tree, Wine Berry,

.... European Walnut

Feline Leukemia .... Common Juniper, Lithy Tree,

.... Rowan Tree

Fibrillation .... European Alder, European

.... Hawthorn

Flatulence .... Fig Tree, European Walnut

Fleas .... Common Juniper, Walnut,

.... Black Currant

Fly Strike.................... Common Juniper, Walnut

Hematoma (post-trauma)

.... Bloodtwig Dogberry, Fig Tree

Heart.......................... European Hawthorn, Maize,

.... European Alder, Red Alder

Heartworm.................Common Juniper, Hawthorn,

.................................European Ash, Black Currant,

.................................European Olive, Common Lilac,

.................................Walnut

Hepatitis ....Common Juniper, Silver Birch,

.................................Common Birch, Rosemary

.................................Rye Grain

Hip Dysplasia ....Common Birch, Wild Woodvine

Hives ....European Alder, Black Currant,

.................................Mountain Pine

Hyperactivity..............Lime Tree

Hypertension ....European Hawthorn,

.................................European Olive, Black Currant,

.................................Lime Tree

Hypothyroidism...........Bloodtwig Dogberry,

.................................Sweet Almond

Hyperthyroidism ....Bloodtwig Dogberry, Lithy Tree

Irritable-Bowel Syndrome

.................................Wine Berry, Fig Tree,

Immune Stimulator..... Briar Rose, European Walnut,

.... Giant Redwood

Immunization detox.... Common Juniper, Black Currant

Infections .... European Walnut, Briar Rose

Inflammation (chronic)

.... European Alder, Common Birch,

.... Briar Rose, European Grape Vine

Injury........................... Black Currant, Common Birch

Insect Bites .... Common Juniper, Black Currant

Insomnia .... Lemon, Lime Tree

Insulin Balancer .... European Walnut

Intervertebral Disc Disease

.... Mountain Pine, Common Birch,

.... Oak, European Beech,

.... Briar Rose, Blackberry Vine

Intestinal parasites..... Fig Tree, European Walnut

Irritability .... Lime Tree

Itching .... Black Currant

Joints..........................Blackberry Vine, Giant Redwood,

..................................Wild Woodvine, Wine Berry,

..................................Mountain Pine, European

..................................Grape Vine

Kennel Cough.............European Filbert, Lithy Tree,

..................................Fig Tree, European Walnut

Keratoconjunctivitis sicca (Dry Eye)

..................................Common Juniper, Black Currant

Kidney drainer ....Silver Birch, Maize,

..................................European Ash, Common Juniper

Kidney insufficiency....European Olive, European Beech

Kidney oxalocalcic stones

..................................Common Juniper, Wine Berry

Kidney stones.............White Birch, Common Juniper,

..................................Black Honeysuckle

Liver Drainer...............White Birch, European Ash,

..................................Common Juniper, Lemon

..................................Rosemary, Rye Grain

Lung Drainer .... European Filbert, Lithy Tree,

.... Maize

Lymphatic Drainer...... European Chestnut

Lyme's Disease .... Briar Rose, European Walnut,

.... Giant Redwood

Mastitis...................... Common Juniper, Mistletoe,

.... European Olive,

.... Rowan Tree

Mast-Cell inhibitor ...... Cedar of Lebanon

Memory...................... European Alder, Rosemary

Metabolism Stimulator Black Currant

Mouth ulcers .... European Alder, Black

.... Honeysuckle

Mucosa, digestive ..... Fig Tree, Wine Berry

Mucosa, inflammation Fig Tree, European Alder,

.... Briar Rose, Lime Tree

Nephritis.................... Common Juniper, Wine Berry,

.... Blackberry Vine,

.... Silver Birch, European Beech

Neutered dogs ....Oak

Obsessive Compulsive Disease

.................................European Olive, Rosemary,

.................................Sweet Almond

Obstructive Respiratory Disease

.................................Blackberry Vine, European Filbert

Osteomyelitis (bone infection)

.................................Red Spruce, European Alder,

.................................Silver Birch

Osteoporosis ....White Birch, Mountain Pine,

.................................Black Currant, Giant Redwood

Pain relief ....Blackberry Vine, Giant Redwood,

.................................Wine Berry, Rowan Tree,

.................................Lime Tree, Mountain Pine

Pancreatic insufficiency

.................................European Walnut

Panic Attacks..............Mistletoe

Parturition (whelping)

.................................Raspberry

Parvo (Canine)........... Fig Tree, Hawthorn, Wine Berry,

.... Briar Rose

Peritonitis .... European Alder

Phobias...................... European Olive, Sweet Almond,

.... Lime Tree

Pituitary stimulations .. Black Currant, Oak

Polyarthritis .... Common Juniper

Prostatitis .... Giant Redwood, Rosemary,

.... Wine Berry

Pulmonary Fibrosis .... European Filbert, Wine Berry

Pulmonary Edema ..... European Hawthorn

Pyometra .... Wine Berry, Briar Rose,

.... Raspberry

Renal Amyloidosis ..... Sweet Almond

Renal Insufficiency..... European Olive, European

.... Beech, Holly Tree

Restlessness .... Lime Tree

Retained Placenta ..... Raspberry

Rhinitis...................... European Alder, Briar Rose

Ringworm ....Rye Grain, Prim Wort,

...................English Elm

Sarcoidosis.................Grape Vine

Sarcoptic mange ....European Alder, Black Currant.

Sclerosis, kidney ....European Beech, Holly Tree

Skin drainer ....Prim Wort, English Elm

Skin Inflammation.......Black Currant

Skin Repair.................Rye Grain

Sneezing ....Briar Rose

Spayed dogs and cats

...................Wine Berry

Spondylitis ....Mountain Pine, Briar Rose,

...................Blackberry Vine

Sprain ....Wild Woodvine

Stress ....Fig Tree, Black Honeysuckle,

...................Lime Tree

Stroke ....European Alder, European Olive,

...................Lime Tree

Synovial inflammation European Ash

Tachycardia .... Hawthorn

Tendon Repair .... Wild Woodvine, Mountain Pine

Tendonitis .... Common Juniper

Teeth (loose) .... Common Birch, Oak

Thrombin-formation regulator

.... Tamarisk

Thrombocytopenia ..... Tamarisk

Thrombosis .... Hedge Maple, European Alder,

.... Red Alder, Common Birch,

.... Red Bud, Bloodtwig Dogberry

.... Hawthorn, Sweet Almond

Thymus regulator .... Fig Tree

Thyroid adenoma .... Wine Berry

Thyroid hyperactive ... Lithy Tree, Bloodtwig Dogberry

Thyroid hypoactive ..... Sweet Almond, Bloodtwig

.... Dogberry

Tinnitus .... Rowan Tree, Lithy Tree,

.... Prim Wort, Mistletoe

Toxicity from drugs (medications)   Black Currant

Tracheitis...................Red Alder, Black Poplar,

.................................Briar Rose,

.................................Lithy Tree, Hornbeam

Trauma......................Wild Woodvine

Tumors, growth inhibitors

.................................Grape Vine, Mistletoe

Ulcers GI ....European Alder, Fig Tree

Ulcerative Colitis.........English Elm, Wine Berry,

.................................Fig Tree

Upper Respiratory ......European Filbert, Lithy Tree,

.................................Briar Rose

Urea (elevated)...........White Birch, Silver Birch,

.................................Common Birch,

.................................Sweet Almond, Mistletoe,

.................................English Elm, Wine Berry

Urethral obstruction (in male cats)

.................................Common Juniper, Black Currant

Urinary infection ....White Birch, Lime Tree,

.................................Wine Berry

Vaccination detoxification

.... Common Juniper,

.... European Alder, Black Currant

Vaginal discharge (leukorrhea)

.... Wine Berry

Vertigo .... Rowan Tree, Lithy Tree,

.... Prim Wort, Rosemary

Vomiting..................... Fig Tree, Grape Vine

Warts .... Fig Tree, Briar Rose, Grape Vine

Wheezing................... European Ash, Black Currant

Worms .... European Ash, Walnut,

.... Black Currant, European Olive

.... Common Lilac

Wounds...................... Black Popular, Raspberry,

.... English Elm, Black Currant

Most Frequently Used Gemmotherapy Remedies in the Care of Animals

- Black Currant
- Black Poplar
- Bloodtwig Dogberry
- Briar Rose
- Cedar of Lebanon
- Common Birch
- Common Juniper
- English Elm
- English Hawthorn
- European Alder
- European Grape Vine
- European Oak
- European Olive
- European Walnut
- Fig Tree
- Giant Redwood
- Hedge Maple
- Lime Tree
- Lithy Tree
- Mountain Pine
- Prim Wort
- Raspberry
- Rosemary
- Rowan Tree
- Rye Grain
- Silver Birch
- Wild Woodvine
- Wine Berry

Resources

Gemmotherapy Remedies & Kits
http://thepetwhisperer.com/healthtips/gemmotherapy

Boiron
http://www.boironusa.com/
(ONLY DOCTORS CAN ORDER FROM THIS SITE)

Gemmotherapy Books

Concentrated Plant Stem Cells-Detoxifications, Regulation, Rejuvenation and Nutrition Professional Guide by Dr. Dominique Richard HMD, ND

*Dynamic Gemmotherapy,***Integrative Embryonic Phytotherapy** by Dr. Joe Rozencwajg, NMD

Gemmotherapy and Oligotherapy Regenerators of Dying Intoxicated Cells, Tridosha of Cellular Regeneration, By Dr. Marcus Greaves M.D.,N.M.D.

Homeopathic Books

Minimum Price Books
http://www.minimum.com/

Homeopathic Remedies & Kits

Washington Homeopathic
www.homeopathyworks.com

Healthy Pet Foods

Bones and Raw Food Diet
http://www.thepetwhisperer.com/products/raw-food

Colostrum

100% New Zealand Bovine Colostrum
http://thepetwhisperer.com/health-tips/colustrum

Essential Oils

Young Living Essential Oils
http://www.thepetwhisperer.com/products/essential-oils

Web sites

www.thepetwhisperer.com

Dr. Blake's website for natural health care for all of your animal friends and their humans. You can also sign up for his free newsletter and learn about the products he recommends for all of your family's natural health care. **This is the site to order your GEMMOTHERAPY remedies, as well as Dr. Blake's books.**

www.AWay2BetterHealth.com

Pam Fettu's website for Gemmotherapy and Homeopathic Health Care for the humans in your animal's life.

www.animalwellnessmagazine.com and www.equinewellnessmagazine.com

Animal Wellness Magazine. Excellent monthly publication on natural products and care of animals from Canada.

www.whole-dog-journal.com

Whole Dog Journal. Another excellent monthly publication on natural care of animals and issues concerning the health of the animals from the United States

Bovine colostrum

http://thepetwhisperer.com/health-tips/colustrum

Source for 100% New Zealand Bovine Colostrum and many other wonderful products for you and your pets. You can order it from this web site, along with other wonderful products for help promote optimum cell replication.

www.colostrumresearch.org

Research site on New Zealand Bovine Colostrum provided for by New Image Inc. Auckland, New Zealand. Excellent research site for information from around the world. Bovine Colostrum is by far the most exciting discovery I have made in the past 37 years. For more information on Bovine

Colostrum The Forgotten Miracle, go
http://www.sedonapurepets.com or
email Joseph.Busuttil@sedonapurepets.com
to learn about this incredible nutritional
supplement.

http://www.mercola.com/

Excellent web site for current health issues
and natural health care for everyone.

Organizations

www.theavh.org
Academy of Veterinary Homeopathy site for
promoting and teaching the practice of
classical (Hahnemannian) homeopathy by
veterinarians

www.drpitcairn.com
Dr. Richard Pitcairn. List of Homeopathic
Veterinarians who have been trained under
Dr. Richard Pitcairn. Site for teaching
veterinarians how to practice classical
(Hahnemannian) homeopathy. Dr. Blake
was in the first class of graduating
homeopathic veterinarians and is certified

under Dr. Pitcairn's course of instruction in classical veterinary homeopathy.

www.AHVMA.org
American Holistic Veterinary Medical Association. This is an organization of which Dr Blake is a founding member and its sole purpose is to support the many holistic methods of alternative veterinary medicine, which include (but are not limited to) homeopathy, chiropractic, acupuncture and nutrition. The organization maintains a list of holistic veterinarians.

http://homeopathic.org/
National Center for Homeopathy. Organization for getting information about homeopathy, monthly journal and list of homeopathic practitioners.

http://www.animalchiropractic.org
American Veterinary Chiropractic Association site for learning more about veterinary chiropractic and how to locate a veterinarian trained in chiropractic principles.

Homeopathic Supplies and Bach Flowers

http://thepetwhisperer.com/washington.html
Washington Homeopathic Pharmacy, Bach Flowers. Homeopathic books, remedies and home kits.

http://www.homeopathic.com
Homeopathic everything. Access to 100+ free articles on homeopathy plus an online catalog of hundreds of books, tapes, medicines, software, and courses. Owner of Homeopathic Educational Services, Dana Ullman, MPH, author of 10 books on homeopathy and leading spokesperson for the field.

http://thepetwhisperer.com/health-tips/gemmotherapy
Gemmotherapy for pets and people. Find about this amazing system of helping the body detoxify and heal. Basic Gemmotherapy Kit for Cats, Dogs and Horses. Single remedies also available.

http://www.thepetwhisperer.com/products/petstore/
All Natural Pet Store, where you can get everything you ever wanted for your pet and it is all safe.

Natural Diets for Pets

http://www.thepetwhisperer.com/products/raw-food/
The word BARF is an acronym for Biologically Appropriate Raw Food. BARF also stands for Bones and Raw Food. This is a site to learn more about the BARF diet and Dr. Billinghurst's work with raw diets.

http://raw4dogs.com
Good site on how to prepare your own raw diets and learn more about raw food for pets.

Flint River Ranch Cat and Dog Food.

Go to www.thepetwhisperer.com to learn more about this natural diet and how to order healthy pet food.

Halo natural pet products.

Go to www.halopets.com to learn more about natural diets and treats for cats, birds and dogs and how to order.

http://www.petguard.com
Excellent dog and cat food.

Vaccination information

http://truthaboutvaccines.org
Truth about vaccines is a web site to give information on the potential dangers of vaccinations.

www.YourPurebredpuppy.com
Find out how many vaccinations your dog really needs, if any. The guidelines have changed, but many veterinarians aren't telling you that. Get current information on how vaccines really work and their potential dangers to the health of your pet. Quotes by many of Dr. Blake's fellow alternative practitioners from around the country.

www.909shot.com
National Vaccine Information Center, dispelling vaccination myths. It is a site that gives information on the history of vaccinations and the warnings you should be aware of for yourself and animals.

www.vaclib.org
Vaccination Liberation site for establishing individual's right not to vaccinate.

www.vaccinationnews.com
Vaccination News is an excellent site to keep current on the serious problems with vaccines and what you can do to help.

http://www.nccn.net/~wwithin/flu.htm
Check out Dr. Sherri Tenpenny's website on the facts about flu vaccines. She has other links on the subject of the coverup and dangers of vaccinations in humans.

Supplement sources

http://www.animalessentials.com/
Supplier of excellent natural animal supplements. Vitamin, mineral and fatty acid supplements for dogs and cats.

http://www.naturvet@naturvet.com
Supplier of natural animal supplements. Extensive list of natural supplements for dogs and cats.

http://www.Apawthecary.com/
Excellent source of natural herbal formulas for animals. Apawthecary is a planet- friendly company too!

http://www.spsocal.com/
Excellent source of glandular supplements for animals and people. Standard Process is the line of glandulars I have used in practice for over 25 years.

Natural Supplies for Cats and Dogs

http://thepetwhisperer.com/products/fleas
Flea, tick, mites and lice natural control products that smell like cedar, are non-toxic to you, your pet or the environment, and best of all, they work. They kill the eggs, larva and adult parasite.

http://thepetwhisperer.com/products/efac
EFAC, a great natural product for helping with the health of your pet's gums and joints.

http://thepetwhisperer.com/products/jointformula
Vetriscience is a superior company that supplies joint nutritional support for your animals.

http://thepetwhisperer.com/products/supplements
Greg Tilford's excellent sources of natural herbal formulas for animals.

www.rainforesthealing.com
Welcome to Rainforest Healing, a place where you have the opportunity to reach down into the Amazon Rainforest, our

planet's greatest "pharmacy." Great herbal company and caregiver to the Rainforest.

http://thepetwhisperer.com/health-tips/are-micro-chips-safe-and-what-is-your-alternative
Natural Identification for your pets and avoids the dangers of micro-chipping.

http://thepetwhisperer.com/health-tips/cataracts
A safe alternative to cataract surgery for your pets.

Sites for Helping the Animals & Planet Earth

http://www.sarveywildlife.org/
Please check out this wonderful Wildlife rescue web site and see how you can help save our friends the animals. Take time to read the story about a Man and an Eagle. It is a beautiful story that will bring tears of joy to your eyes.
http://www.sarveywildlife.org/Story.aspx?id=7 .

www.dolphins.org
Dolphin Research Center (DRC) is a not-for-profit education and research facility, home to a family of Atlantic bottlenose dolphins and California sea lions. Over half of our family was born at the Center, while the other members either have come to us from other facilities or were collected long ago by previous management.

www.elephants.com
Sanctuary for elephants who need our support and care. To shop and help the elephants go to http://www.elephants.com/merchandisestart.htm. You can also help by shopping at ebay to help raise money to take care of my friends the elephants.

www.savearcticrefuge.org
Save the Arctic National Wildlife Refuge created by Robert Redford. An excellent site for becoming aware of what we can do to save our natural wildlife and environment from destruction.

www.bastis.org
A natural health site that is very informative for both animals and their humans with advice on building the immune system naturally.

www.LindaBlair.com
www.LindaBlairFanClub.com
Join Linda Blair in her efforts to help with the protection of animals. She has put her heart and soul into her crusade to providing a better world for our friends the animals.

www.wylandfoundation.org
Wyland Foundation. Dr. Blake is a big admirer of Wyland and his work. He is one of the best friends the seaworld kingdom has on this planet. Helping his work helps all living things on the planet earth.

www.savethewhales.org
Save the Whales Foundation is a wonderful organization that needs all the help it can get to promote its work to preserve one of man's biggest friends, the whale.

Suggested Reading

Boone, J. Allen. *Kinship with All Life.* San Francisco, California: Harper, 1976.

Coulter, Harris. *Vaccination, Social Violence, and Criminality.* Berkeley, California: North Atlantic Books, 1990.

Day, Christopher. *The Homeopathic Treatment of Small Animals.* London: Wigmore Publications, 1984.

Essential Science Publishing. *Essential Oils Desk Reference.* Essential Science Publishing, 2001.

Frazier, Antra, with Norma Ecroate. *The New Natural Cat: A Complete Guide for Finicky Owners.* New York: Plume/Penguin Books, 1990.

Frost, April and Rondi Lightmark. *Beyond Obedience: Training with Awareness for You and Your Dog.* New York: Harmony Books, 1998.

Greaves, Marcus, MD. *Gemmotherapy and Oligotherapy Regenerators of Dying Intoxicated Cells. Xlibris Corporation 2003.*

Hamilton, Don, DVM *Homeopathic Care for Cats and Dogs.* Berkeley, California: North Atlantic Books.

Herscu, Paul, N.D. *The Homeopathic Treatment of Children.* Berkeley, California: North Atlantic Books, 1991.

Kaminski, Patricia, and Richard Katz. *Flower Essence Repertory.* Nevada City, California: Flower Essence Society, 1994. Book of flower essences including the English Bach Flower remedies as mentioned in my book.

Kaslof, Leslie J. *The Traditional Flower Remedies of Dr. Edward Bach: A Self-Help Guide.* (New Canaan, Conn.: Keats, 1988, 1993)

Levy, Juliette de Bairacli. *Cats Naturally.* London: Faber and Faber, 1991.

Levy, Juliette de Bairacli. *The Complete Herbal Book for the Dog and Cat.* London: Faber and Faber, 1991.

Pitcarin, Richard H. D.V.M., & Susan Hubble Pitcairn. *Natural Health for Dogs and Cats.* Emmaus, Pennsylvania: Rodale Press, 1995.

Richard, Dominique, HMD, ND. *Concentrated Plant Stem Cells- Detoxification, Regulation, Rejuvenation & Nutrition, Professional Guide. Copyright 2006.*

Ross-Williams, Lisa *Down-To-Earth: Natural Horse Care. www.down-to-earthhc.com 2010.*

Rozencwajg, Joe, NMD. Dynamic Gemmotherapy. Integrative Embryonic Phytotherapy. Second Edition 2008. Natura Medica Ltd.

Ruiz, Don Miguel, & Ruiz, Don Jose. *The Fifth Agreement: A Practical Guide to Self-Mastery.* San Rafael, CA: Amber-Allen Publishing, 2009.

Schoen, Allen. *Love, Miracles, and Animal Healing.* New York: Simon and Schuster, 1996.

Schwartz, Cheryl. *Four Paws, Five Directions. A Guide to Chinese Medicine for Cats and Dogs.*

Berkeley, California: Celestial Arts. 1996. Great Guide to the use of Chinese Herbal and Acupressure.

Schwartz, Cheryl, DVM. *Natural Healing for Dogs and Cats A-Z.* Hay House, Inc. 2000.

Shadman, Alonzo J. M.D. *Who is your Doctor and Why.* New Canaan, Connecticut: Keats Publishing, Inc

Tilford, Mary L. Wulff-Tilford & Gregory L. *All You Ever Wanted to Know About Herbs for Pets.* Irvine, California: Bowtie Press, 1999.

www.ingramcontent.com/pod-product-compliance
Lightning Source LLC
Chambersburg PA
CBHW061150220326
41599CB00025B/4434